A Veterinary Practitioner Handbook
Series Edited by Neal King BVSC MRCVS

# TRAUMA MANAGEMENT IN THE DOG AND CAT

**John E. F. Houlton** MA, Vet MB, MRCVS, DVR

*Department of Clinical Veterinary Medicine,
University of Cambridge*

and

**Polly M. Taylor** MA, Vet MB, MRCVS, DVA

*The Animal Health Trust,
Newmarket, Suffolk*

r

**WRIGHT**
Bristol
1987

*Published under the Wright imprint by*
IOP Publishing Limited
Techno House, Redcliffe Way, Bristol BS1 6NX


*British Library Cataloguing in Publication Data*

Houlton, John E. F.
    Trauma management in the dog and cat.
    1. Dogs——Wounds and injuries    2. Cats——
    Wounds and injuries    3. Veterinary critical
    care
    I. Title       II. Taylor, Polly M.
    636.7'08971026       SF991


ISBN 0 7236 0696 X


*Typeset by* Activity Ltd, Salisbury, Wilts

*Printed in Great Britain by* The Bath Press,
Lower Bristol Road, Bath BA2 3BL.

# Preface

The aim of this book is to describe methods and techniques used in the management of trauma which are within the scope of general veterinary practice. Simple but effective procedures are covered which require the minimum of sophisticated equipment. We have deliberately omitted more expensive and specialized techniques. A list of recommended equipment, including suppliers, is given in the appendix.

We are indebted to many colleagues who have allowed us access to clinical material. We are grateful to Janet Littlewood for *Figs.* 8.18 and 8.19, to John Fuller for the illustrations and to Janet Butler and Mark Lee for their photographic assistance.

We acknowledge, with affection, the contribution of the late Robert Walker, whose example and teaching influenced many of the methods described.

We should also like to thank our families for their unfailing patience and support in the preparation of the manuscript.

J. H.
P. T.

# Contents

Chapter 1

# The Emergency Case

## THE INITIAL EXAMINATION

The initial examination of a traumatized animal should be systematic, and a set routine should be followed in order that nothing is overlooked. The information gained from this examination is extremely important as the patient's life depends on accurate assessment of the condition and rational treatment. There may be no opportunity to rectify early mismanagement of the case, so it is important that vital signs are not missed or misinterpreted. Adequate respiratory and cardiovascular function must be maintained, and body temperature and chemistry kept within normal physiological limits.

A case history must be taken, but can, if necessary, be obtained during the initial examination. Questions should be short and not phrased to elicit a biased answer. The time of the last meal or drink, any recent medication and the presence of other disease or abnormality should be noted.

In the severely injured animal the initial examination may have to be performed while immediate life-saving measures are undertaken, but whenever possible the condition of the animal should be thoroughly assessed before any treatment is given.

Hypoxia and haemorrhage are the primary causes of early death in the trauma case and need immediate treatment. Hypoxia may result from one or more of the following conditions:

1. Airway obstruction.
2. Respiratory failure (central, or due to chest injury).
3. Circulatory insufficiency.

1

Other conditions arising after trauma which require immediate attention include:

1. Profound shock (which may be a result of haemorrhage).
2. Coma (due to CNS damage).

The order in which the initial examination is performed is a matter of personal choice, but priority must be given to the cardiovascular and respiratory systems and to the detection and control of haemorrhage. The features listed under General examination and Chest below must be assessed first.

## General examination

| | |
|---|---|
| Take | — the rectal temperature. |
| Observe | — the colour of the mucous membranes. |
| Determine | — the capillary refill time. |
| Assess | — the rate, volume and strength of the femoral pulse. |
| Inspect | — for external haemorrhage, vomitus and other discharge. |
| Assess | — skin tone and integrity. |
| Determine | — the state of consciousness. |

## Chest

| | |
|---|---|
| Count | — the respiratory rate. |
| Assess | — the character of breathing. |
| Inspect and palpate | — for penetrating wounds and rib fractures, for equal movement of both sides of the chest, the position of the cardiac apex beat. |
| Percuss | — for areas of increased resonance of dullness |
| Auscultate | — for heart rate, murmurs, arrhythmias. |
| | — for respiratory sounds. |

## Head and neck

| | |
|---|---|
| Inspect | — for injuries, especially of skull, eyes, mouth, nose. |
| Check | — range of head movement. |
| | — for pain. |

## Abdomen

| | |
|---|---|
| Inspect | — for penetrating wounds. |
| Palpate | — for evidence of pain |

|         |                                          |
|---------|------------------------------------------|
|         | — for evidence of fluid.                 |
|         | — to identify individual organs.         |
| Percuss | — for presence of fluid, air.            |
| Perform | — rectal examination.                    |

### Spine and limbs

|         |                                          |
|---------|------------------------------------------|
| Inspect | — for wounds and obvious deformities.    |
| Palpate | — the temperature of extremities.        |
|         | — for fractures and dislocations.        |

### Nervous system

|        |                                          |
|--------|------------------------------------------|
| Assess | — Cranial and peripheral reflexes.       |
|        | — Limb posture and paralysis.            |
|        | — flaccidity/rigidity.                   |
|        | — ability to stand/walk.                 |

## INITIAL MANAGEMENT OF RESPIRATORY PROBLEMS

If the patient is in respiratory distress, immediate action must be taken to ensure adequate pulmonary ventilation. The airway must be cleared of any blood clots or discharge by swabbing or suction. If it is difficult to maintain a clear airway an endotracheal tube should be inserted and the cuff inflated. This will ensure a patent airway, prevent further aspiration of foreign material and will enable assisted ventilation to be performed if necessary. Brachycephalic animals and those with soft palate problems must certainly be intubated if they show signs of respiratory embarrassment. In the severely depressed animal sedation is unnecessary and a mouth gag is often all that is required to prevent the tube from being bitten. Alternatively, the mouth can be taped shut around the tube using a rubber bung or roll of bandage as a wedge between the teeth. Tracheostomy can be life-saving in cases of upper airway obstruction when attempts to intubate have proved unsuccessful. Fortunately it is not commonly required in small animal practice.

Hypoxia, unless severe, can be difficult to detect, but whenever its existence is suspected administration of oxygen is recommended. Signs commonly associated with poor tissue oxygenation include dyspnoea, changes in the heart rate, altered CNS activity (either drowsiness or restlessness) and cool extremities. Cyanosis, contrary to popular belief, is not a reliable sign.

Oxygen can be given by face mask, nasal catheter or endotracheal tube. Hall's face masks are available in several different sizes to fit both cats and dogs. To prevent carbon dioxide accumulation, the mask should not be forced tightly over the face, and a gas flow rate of at least

4 l/min should be used. A mask is usually quite well tolerated by a sick animal but is of no use if it induces struggling, since this will only increase the oxygen demand.

An intranasal catheter may be used to provide oxygen, but must be abandoned if the animal struggles or attempts to remove the tube.

Animals judged to have poor pulmonary ventilation can be assisted with intermittent positive pressure ventilation (IPPV). Ideally 100 per cent oxygen should be used, but where this is unavailable oxygen-enriched air or air alone may be employed.

IPPV is most satisfactorily performed with the animal intubated. It is possible, however, to use a well-fitting face mask for short periods. It must be held firmly in place, to prevent excessive gas leakage. In these circumstances it is easy to inadvertently fill the stomach with air. If this does occur it should be emptied regularly by a stomach tube.

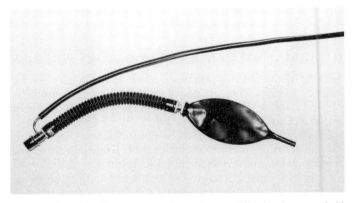

*Fig.* 1.1. An Ayre's T-piece with a Jackson Rees modification (open-ended bag added) can be used to provide IPPV in animals up to 10–15 kg.

IPPV with oxygen is most easily provided by using a suitable breathing circuit supplied from an anaesthetic machine or any oxygen cylinder with a two-stage regulator. An Ayre's T-piece (*Fig.* 1.1) is most suitable for cats and small dogs up to 10 or 15 kg, but a to-and-fro or circle rebreathing system is easier to use in larger dogs. Where no breathing circuit is available an Ambu bag (*Fig.* 1.2) can be used. This is a re-expandable bag with a non-rebreathing valve that can be used to provide IPPV with air when compressed gases are unavailable. Oxygen should be used if at all possible, and in this case is insufflated into the air input of the Ambu bag.

The simplest method by which to gauge adequacy of pulmonary ventilation is by observation of the animal's chest wall. This should move slightly more with each breath than during spontaneous

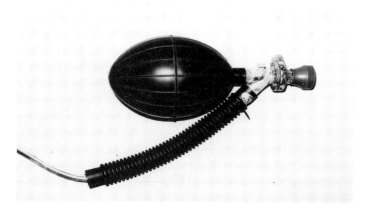

*Fig.* 1.2. An Ambu bag can be used to provide IPPV when a compressed gas supply is unavailable.

respiration. IPPV should not be too vigorous nor too fast or the lungs and circulation may be damaged. Positive pressure in the thorax impedes venous return and therefore depresses cardiac output. This effect can be minimized by employing a short inspiratory period and a longer expiratory pause. In the majority of cases a rate of 10–20 breaths per minute is adequate. In small dogs and cats in particular, an intentional leak in the system (e.g. around the endotracheal tube) will ensure that intrathoracic pressure does not become dangerously high.

## INITIAL MANAGEMENT OF HAEMORRHAGE

External haemorrhage must be controlled by whatever method is appropriate. Clamping or ligation of major vessels may be required, but often a pad and pressure bandage is sufficient as a first line of treatment. Surgery may be required later, once the animal's condition is stabilized. This will depend on the type of wound and the type of blood vessel involved. Arterial haemorrhage is dramatic, but the elasticity of the arterial wall tends to promote blood clotting. Venous haemorrhage is less dramatic but is often the more difficult to control in the long term. If internal haemorrhage is suspected, aspiration from the chest or abdomen will provide a quick and reliable answer.

## INITIAL MANAGEMENT OF CIRCULATORY PROBLEMS

The profoundly shocked animal must receive prompt and vigorous treatment to improve tissue perfusion and prevent deterioration to a

Table 1.1.  Opiate analgesics suitable for use in the dog and cat

| Drug | Dog | Cat |
|------|-----|-----|
| Morphine sulphate (repeat 4 hourly) | 0·2 mg/kg (max 15 mg) | 0·1 mg/kg (max 1 mg) |
| Pethidine hydrochloride (repeat 1–2 hourly) | 2 mg/kg | 2 mg/kg (max 10 mg) |
| Buprenorphine (repeat 6–8 hourly) | 0·01 mg/kg | 0·01–0·03 mg/kg |
| Pentazocine (repeat 6–8 hourly) | 1–2 mg/kg | 1–2 mg/kg |

point where the condition becomes irreversible. A relatively large volume of fluid must be administered quickly, and it is worthwhile catheterizing the jugular vein rather than a peripheral vessel.

## INITIAL MANAGEMENT OF PAIN

This is necessary on humane grounds and may also be physiologically beneficial since pain is likely to contribute to the development of shock. Assessment of pain is a subjective evaluation but analgesia should be provided whenever the existence of pain is suspected. Opiate analgesics are the most effective for relief of acute pain, and when suitable therapeutic doses are given (Table 1.1) the respiratory depression associated with their use is rarely of clinical significance. Indeed, in any condition where breathing is painful, opiate analgesics will actually increase ventilation by enabling the animal to move its chest wall more freely. The opiates may be given by intramuscular or subcutaneous injection, or intravenously if an immediate effect is required. Opiates should not be given if the animal has a head injury since they raise intracranial pressure. This may aggravate any existing cranial pathology.

## ANAESTHESIA OF THE EMERGENCY CASE

It is rarely necessary to anaesthetize the accident case immediately it is presented. There are few injuries that cannot wait until the animal's condition is fully assessed and under control. For instance, it is often wise to defer repair of fractured long bones for 24 or 48 hours, particularly when there has been substantial blood loss and widespread tissue injury. However, there are a number of conditions where immediate surgery is essential in order to save the animal's life. In this case anaesthesia will be required in a possibly shocked and unstable animal, and attention to small detail is essential for the animal's survival.

The emergencies where immediate anaesthesia may be required are:

1. Chest and airway trauma where surgery is required to establish adequate pulmonary ventilation,
2. Haemorrhage, usually internal, which cannot be arrested without surgery,
3. Brain or spinal cord lesions which require decompressive surgery.

In most cases no special equipment or drugs are required for such anaesthesia, but it is essential that no mistakes are made. The traumatized animal does not have the normal reserve of a healthy animal and cannot tolerate, for instance, a period of hypoxia or hypercapnia. Attention to the basic ABC of Airway, Breathing and Circulation covers all the specific needs of the animal.

It is essential that oxygen be used for anaesthesia, even if no inhalation anaesthetic is being used. Oxygen should be given before induction and in the recovery period if possible. In some cases of chest trauma IPPV is life-saving and it is essential that this can be performed as soon as anaesthesia is induced.

In general, smaller doses of all anaesthetic agents will be required. It may be necessary to reduce the induction dose of a barbiturate by up to 50 per cent. The condition of the animal will dictate how much this should be.

An intravenous catheter should be inserted before induction of anaesthesia so that drugs or fluids can be given without delay. It is always much easier to penetrate a vein at an early stage; if the cardiovascular system deteriorates, peripheral vessels collapse, making venepuncture more difficult.

## Anaesthesia for emergency chest and airway surgery

It should be appreciated that there are a number of conditions where the severely dyspnoeic animal improves dramatically once it is anaesthetized, intubated, is breathing oxygen and ventilated by IPPV. For instance, a dog with an open chest wound cannot get air into the collapsed lung by the normal process of inspiration, since the defect in the chest wall allows air to be sucked into the pleural cavity as the chest is expanded (*Fig.* 1.3). As soon as positive pressure is supplied with IPPV, the lung inflates normally, so the wound can be repaired at leisure while IPPV continues. This state of affairs also applies to the flail chest, and in some instances to the tension pneumothorax.

A critical period during anaesthesia is induction. Any increase in oxygen demand, or failure of oxygen to reach the remaining functional lung, may be fatal. Thus induction must be smooth and fast. Intravenous induction is far more satisfactory than a mask induction for

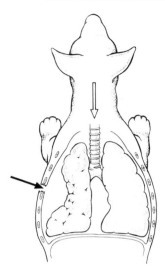

*Fig.* 1.3. An open chest wound causes the ipsilateral lung lobes to collapse on *inspiration* since air is sucked into the pleural cavity.

this reason. Ideally, the animal should be kept in sternal recumbency and must be handled firmly and as sensitively as possible so that no struggling occurs. Premedication may reduce struggling and very small doses (not more than 0·05 mg/kg) of acepromazine may be used with caution in the animal that is not hypovolaemic and is not too depressed. Opiate analgesics are usually more satisfactory premedicants as they make respiration easier and calm the animal through relieving pain. In the acutely dyspnoeic animal there may be no time for premedication, and induction must proceed immediately. Oxygen may be given by mask during induction if it does not cause struggling. Once anaesthesia is induced, intubation is performed immediately, and the animal connected to the breathing circuit. If the animal was having difficulty in inflating its lungs when fully conscious, it should be ventilated with IPPV immediately after induction.

It is advantageous to use neuromuscular blocking agents to facilitate the transfer to IPPV, as these drugs relax all skeletal muscles. In the cat it is preferable to use such drugs before intubation in order to facilitate intubation as well as the transition to IPPV. However, if neuromuscular blocking drugs are not normally used, it is unwise to use them only for accident cases. It is better to become familiar with their use in normal animals.

The recovery period is as important as induction. Hopefully the major problem will have been treated, but since the lungs take some time to re-expand and clear any oedema, the animal will still require support. Oxygen is helpful in this period, but the most significant benefit derives from the use of a chest drain to ensure that all air or fluid is expelled from the pleural cavity. It is not sufficient to inflate the lungs as the last suture closes the thorax, since pockets of air and fluid will be left trapped in the pleural cavity. A chest drain inserted during surgery can be aspirated gently during recovery and for several days after surgery if necessary.

Postoperative analgesia is particularly important after thoracic surgery. Pleural trauma is extremely painful and may cause considerable distress. Recovery will be aided by analgesia, since respiration will be slower and deeper, thus discouraging lung collapse. The animal is also likely to regain an appetite more quickly if it is not in pain.

Surgery of the damaged airway presents different problems, but primarily that of intubation. If intubation can be performed without too much difficulty, there is no further special requirement. However, the recovery period must be carefully monitored, so that any sign of airway obstruction can be dealt with immediately.

If intubation is difficult a tracheostomy should be considered. Once this is performed the animal must be closely monitored until a normal airway is again established.

Airway injuries commonly require careful examination under anaesthesia, even if conservative treatment is indicated. It is most important that these animals are handled carefully, so that struggling does not occur, and that oxygen is available. Induction of anaesthesia must be smooth and fast, and oxygen must be administered, by mask if necessary, as soon as the animal is asleep. The patient should be well oxygenated before any attempt is made to intubate or to examine the airway. Examination or attempts at intubation should be interspersed with periods where the animal is allowed to breathe oxygen from the mask. A tracheostomy must be performed if the airway cannot be adequately maintained by any other method.

### Anaesthesia for surgery to arrest haemorrhage

The main consideration in these cases is that the animal will already have lost a substantial amount of blood and will require fluid therapy. Fluids, preferably partly blood, or at least colloids, should be given as the animal is prepared for surgery, and infusion should continue during surgery and into the recovery period. An intravenous catheter, preferably in a jugular vein, is essential.

Acepromazine premedication should be avoided as this will reduce blood pressure dramatically in the hypovolaemic animal. Opiate premedication is preferable. Doses of intravenous induction agents will be reduced, and as little halothane as possible should be used in order to prevent further hypotension.

## Anaesthesia for CNS surgery

In contrast to the above, in CNS cases it is helpful to produce a degree of hypotension. Acepromazine is a suitable premedicant as long as there is not severe blood loss from other injuries. Opiates should not be used as these increase intracranial pressure and may exacerbate the injury. Over-zealous fluid therapy should be avoided so that cerebral oedema is not enhanced. Diuretics should be given as described in Chapter 5, but care must be taken that the animal does not become dehydrated. An intravenous line should be inserted before anaesthesia is induced so that fluids or other drugs may be given if necessary. Halothane is ideal for CNS surgery as intracranial pressure is reduced.

Chapter 2

# *Shock*

Shock is a clinical syndrome in which there is progressive deterioration of the microcirculation because the cardiovascular system is unable to maintain adequate pressure and flow of blood. Tissues are poorly perfused and the final outcome is hypoxia and cell death. When this is widespread, shock becomes irreversible and the animal dies. It should be emphasized that shock is merely a clinical syndrome and many factors may contribute to its cause; the end result, however, is always failure of the microcirculation and consequent cell damage and death.

It is generally agreed that shock may be caused by any one of the following:

1. Hypovolaemia.
2. Vasodilatation.
3. Myocardial insufficiency.
4. Endotoxins.

**Hypovolaemia**

Hypovolaemic shock results from a decrease in the circulating blood volume. Haemorrhage is the most common cause in the accident case. External haemorrhage may appear dramatic, but the consequences of internal haemorrhage must never be underestimated. Blood lost into the chest may be particularly significant due to the additional effect it will have on impairing respiratory function. A further, often overlooked, source of haemorrhage is within muscle masses at the site of a fracture. However, the degree of shock is related not only to the total volume of blood lost, but also to the rate of loss; therefore the

11

haemorrhage that occurs over several days around a fractured bone is better tolerated than acute haemorrhage incurred when a major vessel is severed. Other causes of hypovolaemia include both 'mixed water and electrolyte' and 'primary water' loss. Mixed water and electrolyte loss is most commonly caused by gastrointestinal disease with vomiting and diarrhoea. Primary water loss is seen as a result of reduced water intake due, for instance, to a fractured jaw. Excessive water loss, as seen with diabetes insipidus, may result in primary water deficiency if there is inadequate drinking water available. Primary water loss rarely causes hypovolaemic shock, whereas a mixed water and electrolyte loss may readily do so. None of these conditions, however, is likely to be a factor in the accident case.

Extensive burns result in considerable fluid loss, but fortunately are not commonly seen in small animals. In these cases the fluid, which has a high protein content, is lost from the surface of the burn by seepage and evaporation. Hypovolaemia may be complicated by toxaemia and infection, resulting in more profound shock than would otherwise be expected from the volume of fluid lost.

The initial response of the body to hypovolaemia is peripheral vasoconstriction mediated by the sympathetic nervous system. This preserves blood supply to vital organs such as the brain and heart. While this is initially life-saving, if it is allowed to continue to extreme, hypoxic cell damage occurs in the areas that are starved of blood flow by the vasoconstriction, and shock ensues.

**Vasodilatation**

Tissue perfusion is dependent on an adequate flow of blood. Stationary or very slow blood flow does not supply sufficient oxygen or remove waste products. As a consequence, inadequate tissue perfusion may result as much from intense vasodilatation as from intense vasoconstriction. Vasodilatation results from loss of sympathetic vascular smooth muscle tone in the arterioles and venules. This may be caused by drugs such as the phenothiazines, by histamine and bradykinin release in anaphylaxis, and in some head and spinal injuries. Even in the absence of true hypovolaemia, the effect of such vasodilatation can be considered as 'effective' hypovolaemia. The volume of blood is unchanged, but now has a much larger vascular bed to fill. Blood pools in the capillary bed, driving pressure is lost and blood flow to the tissues is inadequate for normal function.

Vasodilatation as a cause of shock is most likely to be seen when vasodilators are used in the presence of pre-existing hypovolaemia. Hypovolaemia will have induced a degree of peripheral vasoconstriction to maintain blood pressure and vital blood supply. Peripheral vasoconstriction is abolished by the use of, for instance, aceproma-zine. The reduced blood volume is unable to fill the now enlarged vascular bed, blood pressure falls dramatically, blood flow becomes inadequate throughout the body and shock is the result.

Acepromazine and other vasodilators (such as those used to reduce the afterload in heart failure) should thus be avoided in the presence of suspected hypovolaemia. Sympathetic handling and the judicious use of analgesics will reduce the likelihood of vasodilatation, due to vasovagal syncope, being induced by pain or fright.

## Myocardial insufficiency

Cardiogenic shock occurs when blood flow to the tissues is insufficient because the heart is unable to maintain an adequate cardiac output. It is unusual in animals, unlike the situation in man where myocardial failure due to coronary artery occlusion is relatively common. Inadequate cardiac output may develop as a result of either reduced filling or reduced emptying. Cardiac tamponade caused by haemorrhage into the pericardial sac will reduce cardiac filling. This is often the result of direct trauma, although it may occur spontaneously. Cardiac emptying is insufficient in the presence of myocardial hypoxia and severe dysrhythmias. Myocardial depressant drugs such as halothane may precipitate cardiogenic shock when there is pre-existing myocardial damage.

## Endotoxins

Endotoxins are lipopolysaccharides found in the cell wall of Gram-negative bacteria and have been shown experimentally to induce a state of shock. Their precise role in the clinical syndrome is still under debate, but they are probably most significant in the later stages of shock. There is a large pool of Gram-negative organisms within the normal gastrointestinal tract, and it appears that when hypoxic cell damage reduces the resistance of the intestinal mucosa endotoxins are absorbed and endotoxaemia develops.

Endotoxins have deleterious effects on many parts of the body. One of the major effects is to reduce vascular tone, particularly venous tone, resulting in pooling of blood, reduced venous return and a consequent fall in cardiac output. Arteriolar vasoconstriction is the response, exacerbating that already present and compounding the already existing state of shock. Complement is activated, so that leucocytes adhere to one another and to the endothelium. Lysosomal enzymes are released and capillary permeability is increased.

The development of endotoxaemia therefore hastens the deterioration of body function and undoubtedly contributes to the development of so-called 'irreversible shock', where so much cell damage and circulatory disruption has occurred that no amount of treatment appears able to restore normal function.

## PATHOPHYSIOLOGY OF SHOCK

Although shock may be the result of several different pathological processes, the final pathway is common to all. Hypovolaemia is the most common and comprehensible cause of shock in animals, and a description of the development of hypovolaemic shock is given below. Other causes of shock are discussed in relation to it.

The body responds to hypovolaemia by peripheral vasoconstriction of arterioles due to sympathoadrenal stimulation. This protects the arterial side of the circulation and reduces capillary pressure. Reduction in capillary pressure leads to an increased reabsorption of extracellular fluid which boosts the circulating blood volume. The venous side of the circulation is also affected, and venule tone increases, thereby increasing venous return and cardiac output. Contraction of the spleen forces reserve erythrocytes into the circulation, further boosting the circulating volume. When, in spite of these measures, blood volume is still inadequate, supply to the vital areas, namely the brain and the heart, is maintained at the expense of the rest of the body.

In the short term, the above measures are life-saving. A loss of 35 per cent of the circulating blood supply can generally be compensated for in the healthy animal, but a loss of 50 per cent is usually fatal without treatment. The blood volume of a dog is approximately 88 ml/kg, thus a blood loss of 400 ml from a 10 kg dog is life-threatening.

It is the exacerbation of the protective mechanisms that leads to shock. Arteriolar vasoconstriction leads to the development of ischaemic hypoxia in the capillary endothelium and the surrounding tissues. Oxygen is in short supply, so energy production by the less efficient anaerobic metabolism takes place. The resulting build-up of lactic and pyruvic acid further damages the local tissue. The endothelium loses its integrity and fluid leaks back into the extracellular spaces. Blood viscosity increases, and blood flow decreases yet further due to sludging and the formation of microthrombi. The situation is worsened by pooling of blood in the capillaries due to maintenance of venous tone while arteriolar tone relaxes in the presence of toxic waste products. Capillary pooling results in more fluid loss through the leaky capillary wall, and the situation is compounded.

The final result is that metabolic wastes accumulate, acidosis develops and cells become short of energy supplies. The integrity of the cell membrane is lost and the sodium pump fails. Cells take up sodium and water and lose potassium. Cellular oedema develops, further compromising cellular function; lysosome and mitochondrial function is also affected, and damage to lysosomes results in the loss of enzymes into the cytoplasm, which further damages the cell.

Hypoxia and acidosis are detrimental to all tissues, but the effect on the myocardium is particularly significant. Cardiac output falls further, and a vicious cycle of deteriorating blood flow and failing cellular function develops (*see Fig. 2.1*).

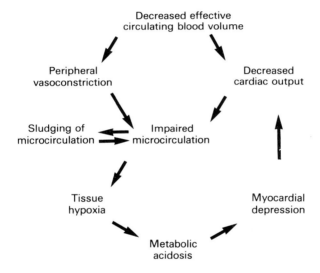

*Fig.* 2.1. Vascular changes in hypovolaemic shock.

The early stage of vasoconstriction may not be seen in true vasodilatory shock, where pooling of blood in the periphery is the major problem, although there may be intense arteriolar vasoconstriction where venous pooling predominates. This state of affairs is most likely to be seen in endotoxic shock where endotoxins compound the deterioration by contributing to the intravascular and endothelial changes.

The most significant effects of circulatory failure are on the kidney, the liver and the intestine. The brain and heart suffer less as the circulatory changes are geared to maintaining their blood supply at the expense of the rest of the body. Skin and muscle also become ischaemic, but the consequences are relatively insignificant in comparison with the effects on kidney, liver and gut. Substantial quantities of the products of anaerobic metabolism may, however, be flushed from muscle tissue into the circulation once the circulation is restored.

The kidneys receive approximately 25 per cent of the cardiac output, and are very susceptible to decreased blood flow caused by hypotension and hypovolaemia. Glomerular filtration ceases once arterial blood pressure falls below 65 mmHg, and if a poor blood supply or total ischaemia persists for a comparatively short period of time (90 minutes in man), acute renal failure develops.

The liver normally functions under relatively hypoxic conditions because much of its blood supply is portal blood. In this respect it has little reserve and hepatic hypoxia probably develops early in the course of shock. In the dog in particular this allows proliferation of anaerobic bacteria and toxin production. Energy metabolism is also affected, and the reticuloendothelial system is severely altered so that phagocytosis and detoxification are curtailed.

The canine small intestine is particularly susceptible to haemorrhagic necrosis as a result of hypoxic damage. This leads to breakdown of the normal barrier to absorption, and toxic products from the bowel lumen can reach the bloodstream.

The clinical signs of shock are outlined in *Table 2.1*.

## TREATMENT OF SHOCK

**Fluid administration**

There is little doubt that of all the measures available, fluid therapy is the most beneficial. The aim is to restore an adequate circulating blood volume so that all tissues are perfused. The type of fluid required, the amount and the rate of administration are important, since inappropriate fluid or inadequate quantity may not produce the desired result.

The choice of fluid will depend upon what is available and economics, but certain criteria must be met:

1. The fluid should be retained in the vascular space for a reasonable period of time to re-establish the circulating blood volume, and must be safe to give rapidly in large quantities. Crystalloid fluids suffer from the disadvantage that only 20–25 per cent of that administered is retained within the circulation after 30 minutes, with the remainder being redistributed in the interstitial spaces and excreted by the kidneys. Very large volumes of crystalloids are therefore needed to maintain the circulating blood volume. Moreover, development of oedema is a potential hazard because of the

Table 2.1. **Clinical signs of shock**

| System | Sign | Condition |
|---|---|---|
| | Subnormal temperature (variable in septic and endotoxic shock) | |
| Skin | Cold extremities | Peripheral vasoconstriction |
| | (Warm extremities in vasodilatory shock) | |
| GI tract | Frequent defecation followed by stasis | ↓ splanchnic blood flow |
| | Blood-tinged faeces in endotoxic shock | Mucosal slough |
| Urinary system | Oliguria or anuria | ↓ glomerular filtration rate |
| Respiratory system | ↑ respiratory rate | Metabolic acidosis |
| Cardiovascular system | ↓ pulse strength and volume | Fall in cardiac output and arterial blood pressure |
| | ↑ pulse rate | Tachycardia due to hypovolaemia |
| | (Bradycardia in terminal stages of shock) | |
| | (May have reasonable pulse volume in endotoxic and septic shock) | |
| | (Superficial veins engorged in cardiogenic shock) | |
| Mucous membranes | Pale cold clammy | Peripheral vasoconstriction |
| | Cyanotic | Hypoxia |
| | ↑ capillary refill time | Poor peripheral perfusion |
| | (Pink and warm in any vasodilatory shock) | Peripheral vasodilatation |
| Sympathetic system | Pupillary dilatation restlessness, shivering | Sympathetic stimulation |
| CNS | Depression and coma | Cerebral hypoxia |

redistribution of these• fluids. This can be avoided by careful monitoring of the patient. Undertransfusion is a far more common mistake than overtransfusion, but a degree of caution is required in patients with pulmonary, renal or cardiac damage, or where cerebral oedema is suspected, since fluid overload may be fatal in such cases.

2. The fluid should be isotonic and thus result in no net movement of water into or out of cells. Hypotonic solutions, such as 0·18 per cent saline or 5 per cent dextrose, when given in large volumes, could cause cellular oedema. Even if this does not occur, such fluid is rapidly lost from the circulation.

3. The fluid should be isoionic, i.e. its ionic concentration should be comparable with that of the extracellular fluid. The ionic losses in shock are generally associated with blood loss, and although electrolyte shifts do occur between body compartments, these are generally due to redistribution rather than actual loss of one ion.

4. The fluid should be close to a normal pH since excessively acidic or alkaline solutions will place unreasonable demands on the body's buffer system. It may be necessary to treat the metabolic acidosis that develops in shock but this is often unnecessary since the body's own homeostatic mechanisms will function again once tissue perfusion is restored.

5. The fluid should be non-toxic and non-immunogenic so that repeated transfusions do not induce an immune response.

6. The fluid should not interfere with the administration of blood as it may be necessary to use this to supplement crystalloid or colloid fluids.

7. The fluid should not influence coagulation or haemostasis.

8. The fluid should be reasonably priced and easily stored.

### Crystalloid fluids

Of the crystalloid fluids available, lactated Ringer's solution comes nearest to satisfying the above criteria. It may seem undesirable to infuse lactate when there is already a lactic acidosis. However, lactate is a bicarbonate precursor, and it has been demonstrated that once hepatic perfusion is restored by fluid administration, the liver is easily able to metabolize the lactate and lactated Ringer's proves to be a rational method of treating the acidosis.

Normal saline (0·9 per cent) is isotonic but it is inferior to lactated Ringer's since it is not isoionic. Hypotonic solutions such as 0·18 per cent saline and 5 per cent dextrose should not be used because of the danger of water intoxication.

Crystalloid fluids should be administered as rapidly as possible in the profoundly shocked animal, and there is little place for a small needle in the cephalic vein. Jugular catheterization involves little extra time and this is soon repaid since it can be used to monitor central venous pressure. In the dog an initial volume of 80 ml/kg may be given in the first hour while 50 ml/kg is a reasonable volume in the cat. Following this initial 'loading volume' the effective circulating blood volume should be reassessed, and in most cases the rate of infusion can now be reduced. It is not unusual for 200 ml/kg to be required (i.e. twice the normal circulating blood volume) as the capillary beds will be dilated and need to be perfused.

The packed cell volume and plasma protein concentration will be markedly reduced after infusions of large volumes of crystalloid fluids have been given. This is likely to be beneficial, since it will tend to counteract the effects of sludging and intravascular coagulation. However, hypoproteinaemia and to a lesser extent low haemoglobin concentration may become a limiting factor in the use of crystalline fluids alone. The safe lower limits of haemodilution are a PCV of 20 l/l and plasma protein of 35 g/l; should either fall below these values, blood, plasma or plasma replacement fluids (colloid) should be given.

### Colloid fluids

Blood and plasma may not be available in practice, but plasma replacement fluids offer an alternative source of colloid fluid that is easily obtained and stored. Due to their higher molecular weight, colloid solutions are retained within the circulation for a longer period than crystalloid fluids.

A degraded gelatin product (Haemaccel, Hoechst) is undoubtedly the most useful colloid solution for use in dogs and cats. Dextrans are also available, and the use of Dextran 70 (containing dextrans of a molecular weight of 70,000) has been quite successful, although the occasional abberant reaction occurs.

Haemaccel is made up in a balanced electrolyte solution and has a half-life of 2–5 hours, after which it is excreted by the kidney. It has an oncotic pressure comparable to plasma and can be used on its own to increase the circulating blood volume.

Dextrans draw fluid from the extracellular spaces into the circulation, hence they are actually plasma expanders. Crystalloid fluids should be given with dextrans to make up the extracellular losses.

Since colloids remain within the circulation, overtransfusion is a potential hazard. It is advisable that central venous pressure be measured when volumes over 20 ml/kg are infused. If they are used rationally, colloids are most effective in the treatment of shock because they enable the circulating blood volume to be restored more rapidly than if crystalloids are used.

### Plasma and blood

The albumin fraction of plasma is particularly valuable as it counteracts the hypoalbuminaemia that occurs as a result of the loss of albumin through the hypoxic capillary endothelium. However, although it is a more physiological solution than the synthetic plasma substitutes, lack of availability limits its use.

Blood must be used in the treatment of severe haemorrhage, but crystalloids in conjunction with colloids are generally preferred in the initial stages of the treatment of shock. If the response to the initial therapy is poor, blood may then be considered. It is important to note that, because of the sludging that occurs in shock, haemodilution is beneficial. Even after severe haemorrhage it is essential to use crystalloids as well as blood in order to decrease blood viscocity and aid blood flow.

Blood may be collected for storage from both dogs and cats. It should be collected into citrate phosphate dextrose adenine (CPD-A) under aseptic conditions. It can be stored in the refrigerator for up to one month. It is most convenient to use blood bags designed for human use for collection from dogs. In the cat a 30 ml syringe containing 5 ml CPD-A (e.g. drawn from a human blood collecting bag) is more practical. The jugular vein is the most suitable vein for collection from both species.

After 1 month's storage the plasma can be harvested, preferably after centrifugation. It can be stored frozen for up to 6 months. If no suitable centrifuge is available, some plasma can be obtained if the red cells are allowed to sediment in the base of the bag. It should be noted that plasma harvested in this way will not contain clotting factors.

## Oxygen therapy

Oxygen administration will raise the blood oxygen tension and thus aid the treatment of tissue hypoxia. Assisted ventilation is rarely required, and in most cases oxygen can be adequately administered by face mask or nasal tube.

## Body temperature

A shivering animal uses energy that it can ill afford, and body heat must be conserved by insulation. Body temperature should not be raised too rapidly or the resulting vasodilatation will be detrimental. Replacement of the circulating blood volume in a shocked animal will in itself do much to raise a subnormal temperature, but fluids, especially if given rapidly, must be pre-warmed to body temperature.

The animal should be warmed by placing it on heating pads and by wrapping it in insulating material such as blankets or plastic packing material (*Fig.* 7.2). Heating pads and hot water bottles that are uncomfortably hot to hold will burn an unconscious animal and must not be used. Warming by insulation is safer and is normally far more effective.

## Antibiotics

All shock cases should be given antibiotic cover to protect against bacterial proliferation. Broad spectrum bactericidal antibiotics such as ampicillin should be injected intravenously to achieve rapid blood levels. The use of metronidazole (Torgyl, May and Baker) may be considered in the treatment of endotoxic shock to combat the release of anaerobes from the bowel.

## Corticosteroids

The use of corticosteroids in the treatment of shock is still controversial, but it is generally agreed that they improve tissue perfusion by improving myocardial contractility and by reducing peripheral vasoconstriction. To be effective steroid administration must begin as soon as possible, and pharmacological rather than therapeutic doses must be used. Hydrocortisone and methylprednisolone have a rapid onset of action and are the drugs of choice. Dexamethasone has a slower onset but its effects are more prolonged. Recommended dosages are given in *Table* 2.2.

*Table 2.2.* **Corticosteroids in shock**

| | |
|---|---|
| Methyl prednisolone | 30 mg/kg i.v. infusion over 30 min |
| Hydrocortisone | 50 mg/kg i.v. over 2–3 min, may repeat hourly |
| Dexamethasone | 5–10 mg/kg i.v. over 2–3 min, repeat in 8 h |

Corticosteroids should not be used in shock unless intravenous therapy is under way, since the subsequent vasodilatation will be counter-productive. Few other adverse effects may be expected since the period of therapy is insufficient to suppress the adrenal cortex.

### Drugs acting on the cardiovascular system

#### *Catecholamines*

Sympathomimetic drugs have been used to raise and maintain arterial blood pressure by utilizing their vasoconstricting properties. However, since tissue perfusion is of paramount importance and peripheral vasoconstriction has already been initiated, these drugs should be used with extreme caution. They may, however, be useful in the circumstances outlined below (*Table* 2.3 gives recommended dosages):

(i) As an emergency measure in severe hypotension and true vasodilatory shock before fluid therapy can be instituted. The smallest

Table 2.3. *Drugs acting on the cardiovascular system*

| | |
|---|---|
| Dopamine | 5–20 µg kg$^{-1}$ min$^{-1}$ i.v. |
| Dobutamine | As for dopamine |
| Adrenaline | 1:10 000 1–5 ml i.v., intracardiac |

dose necessary to maintain a reasonable (not normal) blood pressure should be used to protect the cerebral and cardiac circulation.

(ii) Where circulatory collapse is imminent and all other measures have failed.

(iii) Where myocardial support is required. This is discussed in Chapter 7.

## Vasodilators

Vasodilators such as the phenothiazines (of which acepromazine is one) may be used to improve tissue perfusion, but they must only be used in conjunction with intravenous fluid replacement. Used on their own they will exacerbate the effects of shock by causing severe hypotension.

## Correction of metabolic acidosis

Measurement of the acid-base status is not a practical proposition without the use of sophisticated equipment, although measurement of urinary pH may provide some evidence of metabolic acidosis. Since the imbalance is secondary to poor tissue perfusion it is safer to correct the primary cause than to attempt correction of the acidosis by the administration of alkali. However, if the condition is severe or the patient unresponsive to treatment, intravenous sodium bicarbonate (2–4 mmol (mEq)/kg for each 30 min shock) may be given. Careful monitoring is required, for excess bicarbonate can cause an increase in intracellular potassium concentration and induce cardiac dysrhythmias.

Treatment of shock is summarized in *Table 2.4*.

## MONITORING DURING SHOCK THERAPY

(See also the section on monitoring in intensive care in Chapter 7.) Physical examination of the animal can be augmented with the use of some laboratory investigations. The value of recording simple clinical signs should not be underestimated, but single measurements are of relatively little value and recording should be carried out at regular intervals so that response to treatment can be assessed objectively.

*Table 2.4.* **Summary of shock treatment**

---

1. Catheterize jugular vein and obtain baseline blood sample
2. Begin rapid infusion of crystalloid fluid or Haemaccel i.v.
3. Give 30 mg/kg methyl prednisolone by i.v. infusion
4. Give ampicillin (5–7 mg/kg)
   Consider the use of metronidazole (20 mg/kg per day by infusion) in endotoxic shock
5. Catheterize bladder and monitor urinary output
6. Monitor temperature, respiratory rate, capillary refill time, femoral pulse and CVP every 30 min
7. Maintain body temperature above 35° C (94° F)
8. If poor response, consider plasma or blood. Maintain PCV between 20 and 45 l/l

---

## Temperature

Body temperature provides a useful guide to prognosis in the treatment of shock. A subnormal temperature that rises carries a good prognosis, but if the temperature falls further, the outlook is poor. The temperature of the extremities can be assessed by palpation. They will be cold where there is severe peripheral vasoconstriction, but may be warm when peripheral vasodilatation has occurred, as in endotoxic shock and septicaemia.

## Pulse

Changes in pulse rate and quality provide a useful means of assessing response to treatment and prognosis. A stronger, slower pulse indicates a favourable response to treatment, whereas a fast and thready pulse is a poor sign. Return of a palpable peripheral pulse is a favourable sign and is also a comparatively objective assessment.

## Respiration

Changes in respiratory rate and pattern provide some information about the response of the patient to treatment of shock; an increased rate is often the first sign of hypoxia. Auscultation should be performed regularly as fluid râles may be the first sign of overtransfusion.

## Capillary refill and mucous membrane colour

Capillary refill time gives a rough guide to the peripheral perfusion. A slow refill (greater than 2 s) indicates that perfusion is poor, but a normal refill time may be seen when there is capillary pooling and equally poor perfusion. This examination must be interpreted in the light of other clinical signs.

### Packed cell volume and plasma protein

Packed cell volume (PCV) and plasma protein (PP) concentration are of limited value in the diagnosis of shock but can be used to monitor the patient's progress and to assess the type of fluid required. A 'baseline' blood sample should be taken before treatment begins and then regular samples taken as therapy progresses.

Interpretation of PCV alone may be difficult, as pre-existing anaemia (low PCV) or dehydration (high PCV) will confuse the picture. The PCV will fall after severe haemorrhage, as interstitial fluid moves into the plasma, but this is not instantaneous, and will only become obvious after a few hours. Plasma or fluid loss into body compartments such as the intestine or extracellular fluid result in a raised PCV. This is most marked in endotoxic shock where the damaged capillary endothelium allows water, electrolytes and eventually protein to leak into the interstitial space.

Evaluation of the plasma protein concentration gives an assessment of the colloid oncotic pressure, and is, therefore, a useful guide to the type of fluid that should be given.

### Central venous pressure

Central venous pressure (CVP) measurement is particularly valuable during treatment of shock, as it provides an accurate and continuous assessment of the progress of fluid therapy, and of cardiac function.

In hypovolaemic and endotoxic shock the CVP is low, whereas it may be near normal in pure vasculogenic shock. Cardiogenic shock (in the normovolaemic animal) is characterized by a high CVP since the heart is unable to function adequately as a pump, and pressure builds up on the venous side of the circulation.

### Urinary output

This provides an extremely useful assessment of internal perfusion. Kidney function is susceptible to poor perfusion, and urine output ceases when blood flow is insufficient.

Anuria that does not respond to intravenous fluid therapy indicates acute pre-renal failure. This is a consequence of the poor perfusion that occurs in shock, and carries a guarded or poor prognosis.

Chapter 3

# The Respiratory System

Thoracic injuries may cause acute respiratory failure and are a common cause of death in accident victims. Injuries to the larynx and upper airways are less common, but are still significant. It is essential for the animal's survival that such injuries are accurately identified and that appropriate treatment is prompt. Animals with thoracic damage often have other injuries as well, and treatment must not be undertaken without paying due regard to all of these. Nevertheless, alleviation of respiratory distress should take priority over everything other than the control of severe haemorrhage.

The intrathoracic structures are normally well protected by the strong yet resilient rib cage and it requires considerable force to damage them. This force may be from blunt trauma, such as occurs in road traffic accidents, falling from heights, crushing injuries, or when an animal collides with a stationery object. Alternatively, penetrating injuries from stakes and other sharp objects, from dog fights and from gunshot or bullets can cause significant damage to the intercostal tissues and the intrathoracic structures.

It is convenient to classify thoracic injuries according to their effect on the respiratory system:

1. Obstruction or disruption of the upper airways
   tracheal rupture
   tracheal foreign bodies
   laryngeal wounds
2. Disruption of the thoracic wall
   rib fractures/flail chest
   open wounds in the chest wall
   intercostal tears without skin damage

25

3. Impaired alveolar function
     pulmonary contusion
     pulmonary laceration
4. Reduced lung volume due to
     intrapleural air
     intrapleural fluid
     intrapleural viscera (ruptured diaphragm)

Fortunately, despite the often dramatic nature of some of these conditions, successful treatment is relatively simple.

## Principles of management

The aim of emergency treatment is to restore and maintain pulmonary and circulatory function. Initial management should ensure a patent airway, and should restore the integrity of the chest wall. It may be necessary temporarily to plug or cover chest wall defects until the animal's condition is stabilized and surgical repair is feasible. Subsequent treatment includes re-expansion of the lungs by thoracocentesis and ensuring adequate ventilation and oxygenation. Adequate analgesia is an essential part of the management of chest injuries. Chest pain results in fast, shallow breathing which is detrimental to pulmonary function. Analgesia, as well as making the patient more comfortable, improves the respiratory function, sometimes dramatically.

The animal with thoracic injuries may also be suffering from shock, and initial management must include treatment for this. Thoracic injuries commonly associated with shock include tension pneumothorax, severe haemothorax and extensive pulmonary contusion.

Thoracic injuries often occur in combination and there are few pathognomonic signs related to any one condition. A systematic physical evaluation is essential and this should include inspection palpation, percussion and auscultation of the chest (*Table* 3.1). However, the extent of the damage is often only fully appreciated after thorough examination of good quality radiographs. Radiography performed soon after the injury may demonstrate a pneumothorax or haemothorax, but it is often several hours before pulmonary changes are seen. These changes may become more severe over the subsequent 24–48 hours and it is advisable to radiograph the chest once or twice daily if the animal's condition is not improving. It is important to use the same exposure throughout serial examinations so that changes in density may be fully appreciated. For the same reason, radiographs should, where possible, be taken during the same stage of the respiratory cycle. In general, radiographs are taken at full inspiration, but when looking for small amounts of pleural fluid or air, radiographs taken at expiration may be useful.

*Table 3.1.* **Clinical signs associated with chest trauma**

| | Possible significance |
|---|---|
| 1. *Inspection* | |
| Open wounds | Open pneumothorax |
| 2. *Observation* | |
| Rapidly developing dyspnoea | Pneumothorax |
| | Pulmonary contusion |
| Less acute dyspnoea | Haemothorax |
| | Ruptured diaphragm |
| Slowly developing dyspnoea | Chylothorax |
| | Pyothorax |
| Rapid shallow breathing (painful) | Rib fractures |
| Asymmetry of chest wall | Flail chest, intercostal tears |
| 3. *Palpation* | |
| Flail segments | Flail chest |
| Displaced cardiac apex beat | Ruptured diaphragm |
| Intercostal tears | Chest wall rupture |
| Subcutaneous emphysema | Pneumomediastinum, open wound |
| 4. *Percussion* | |
| Hyper-resonance | Pneumothorax |
| Hyporesonance | Haemothorax, chylothorax, pyothorax, ruptured diaphragm |
| 5. *Auscultation* | |
| Râles | Pulmonary haemorrhage |
| Reduced pulmonary sounds | Pneumothorax |
| | Ruptured diaphragm |
| Muffled heart sounds | Haemothorax |
| | Chylothorax |
| Borborygmi | Ruptured diaphragm |
| Cardiac dysrhythmias | Myocardial contusion |

Thoracic radiography must be performed with care so as not to cause further distress by careless handling of the animal. It is particularly important not to roll the animal on to its back. If the animal is turned over, fluid or abdominal contents in the pleural cavity will be forced downwards by gravity, and the *dorsal* lung field will suddenly be compressed. If this occurs, the animal may have very little functional lung available, since the *ventral* lobes will already be compromised.

Oxygen administration is an essential part of the management of thoracic trauma, particularly where alveolar perfusion is adequate but pulmonary ventilation is compromised (as in conditions where there is reduced lung volume due to intrapleural fluid, air or viscera).

Thoracocentesis is commonly employed in the management of thoracic trauma. It can either be used to collect pleural fluid in order to establish its nature, or to remove air or fluid from the pleural space to permit re-expansion of the lungs. If thoracocentesis needs to be

*Table 3.2.* **Indications for thoracotomy**

1. Penetrating thoracic wounds
2. Severe and persistent bleeding
3. Severe and persistent air leak
4. Oesophageal perforation with mediastinal contamination

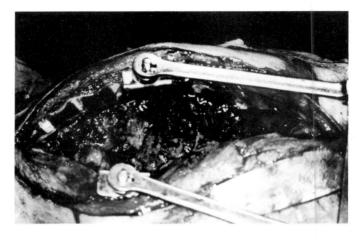

*Fig.* 3.1. A median sternotomy may be more useful than a paracostal incision since it permits greater exposure and better access to the intrathoracic structures. It should be repaired with stainless steel wire sutures passed around each sternebra.

repeated because there is further accumulation of air or fluid, a thoracic drainage tube should be inserted (*see* Chapter 8). The pleural space can then be aspirated continuously or as frequently as necessary. Continued leakage in spite of repeated or continuous drainage necessitates a more aggressive approach, and surgery may be required. In general, however, surgery should only be considered after thoracocentesis and chest tube drainage have failed.

Thoracotomy is not often necessary in the management of thoracic trauma but there are certain conditions where there is no alternative treatment (*Table* 3.2). Unless the precise location of the lesion is known preoperatively, it is wise to open the chest using a median sternotomy ('sternal split') (*Fig.* 3.1). This provides wider exposure of the intrathoracic structures than does a lateral approach and permits fuller appraisal of the damage.

## TRACHEA

**Wounds of the larynx and trachea**

These are usually the result of fights or penetrating wounds of the cervical region.

Dyspnoea may be caused by a breach in the airway, but is more often due to airway obstruction by damaged tissues, haematoma formation or oedema. Subcutaneous emphysema and a pneumomediastinum, with or without a pneumothorax, generally develop rapidly.

The larynx should be examined with the animal anaesthetized (*see* Chapter 1) and the extent of the wound explored. Many injuries will heal spontaneously, although, if there is a significant obstruction or severe swelling, a tracheostomy will be necessary (*see* Chapter 8). Concomitant damage to the pharynx or cranial oesophagus will cause dysphagia, and feeding via a pharyngostomy tube may be required while the injuries heal. Conservative treatment comprises cage rest, thoracocentesis if a pneumothorax is present and broad spectrum antibiotic cover.

Tracheal rupture may be total, or may be incomplete with the dorsal membrane holding the two portions together. The gap may be palpable, or a skin wound may indicate the location of the rupture. Intubation should be attempted, but if it is impossible to slide the tube into the distal portion, a tracheostomy caudal to the rupture is essential. Location of the rupture can be confirmed by endoscopy. Rupture of the thoracic trachea is unusual and may respond to conservative treatment. If this is not successful surgical repair is necessary.

The edges of a tracheal rupture should be débrided and sutured with non-absorbable horizontal mattress sutures. This ensures apposition of the mucosal surfaces and places the knots of the sutures outside the tracheal lumen.

**Tracheal foreign bodies**

Foreign bodies in the form of metallic or vegetable material are unusual, and the common obstructions are blood clots or food material. In the accident case severe epistaxis may result in blood clots occluding the major airways. This is particularly likely in animals that are semi-comatosed or those that have a depressed cough reflex. Nasal and maxillary fractures can be particularly distressing as, apart from causing serious epistaxis, the depressed fracture fragments often occlude the nasal passages as well (*Fig.* 3.2).

Treatment must establish a clear airway and control haemorrhage. Anaesthesia is usually required for these cases, and extreme care must

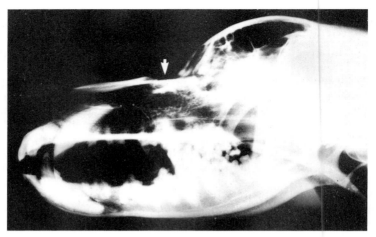

*Fig.* 3.2. Lateral radiograph of a Greyhound's skull showing a depressed fracture of the naso-frontal bones (arrow).

be taken to prevent the airway from being further occluded, particularly at induction. The trachea should be aspirated and intubated, and oxygen should be administered. Ice packs applied over the nose are helpful in controlling epistaxis. The nasal passages can be packed in the unconscious animal, but this is inadvisable in the conscious patient as it provokes further sneezing.

Although beyond the scope of this book, other causes of upper airway obstruction which may present as acute respiratory distress should not be forgotten. These include stenotic nares, elongation of the soft palate, collapse of the arytenoid cartilages and eversion of the lateral cartilages. Laryngeal paralysis in the dog and cat, and laryngospasm in the cat, are further conditions to bear in mind.

## THE RIBS

### Rib fractures

Rib fractures are a common sequel to blunt thoracic trauma and unless associated with other injuries they are often of little clinical significance. However, respiration is painful and the animal is discouraged from coughing. This may occasionally permit the build-up of obstructive bronchial secretions and predispose to pneumonia.

Pain over the affected ribs is evident with or without associated soft tissue swelling and subcutaneous emphysema. The diagnosis is confirmed by radiography.

Treatment of uncomplicated rib fractures is conservative, and healing is usually rapid with cage rest or restricted exercise. Analgesics will permit deeper respiration and make coughing less painful.

Complications of rib fractures include torn intercostal vessels, lacerated lung lobes and pulmonary contusion. A haemothorax or pneumothorax may thus coexist, necessitating thoracocentesis. Surgical stabilization of rib fractures using Kirschner and/or cerclage wires is only required in unusual cases where there is marked displacement and the fractured ribs are liable to cause further damage to the underlying lung.

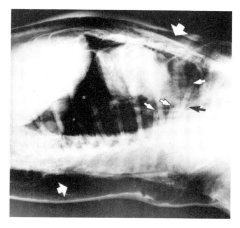

*Fig.* 3.3. Lateral radiograph of a terrier's thorax with multiple rib fractures (small arrows) and subcutaneous emphysema (large arrows).

## Flail chest

Proximal and distal fractures of two or more adjacent ribs (*Fig.* 3.3) may result in a free section of the chest wall that moves paradoxically with respiration. A similar flail segment is mobilized when consecutive ribs of a young animal are fractured proximally (since the costal cartilages are pliable in animals of this age). During inspiration the flail segment will be drawn inward while the rest of the thoracic cage is expanding, and on expiration the reverse movements occur. Dyspnoea is often severe due to the cumulative effect of the paradoxical breathing and the contusion of underlying lung tissue. Flail chest injuries commonly occur when a small dog is picked up and crushed in the jaws of a larger dog.

The diagnosis is made by observation and palpation of the flail segment, and is confirmed by radiography. Initial treatment should stabilize the flail segment to prevent further damage. As emergency

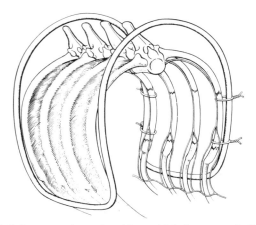

*Fig.* 3.4. A flail segment is produced by multiple fractures of adjacent ribs. It can be immobilized by securing it to a padded aluminium frame contoured to the chest wall. The frame should be secured with stainless steel wire or heavy monofilament nylon. The intercostal vessels which run caudal to each rib should be avoided. The frame may be used both for emergency and longer term treatment.

treatment, the segment can be pulled out with towel clamps applied around the fractured ribs.

The flail segment can be supported by securing the affected ribs to a padded aluminium rod frame contoured to the rib cage (*Fig.* 3.4). Alternatively, the segment can be immobilized by internal fixation of the rib fractures. This is the treatment of choice, particularly where other chest injuries have to be repaired, although surgery may have to be delayed until the animal's condition is stable.

## PNEUMOTHORAX

Pneumothorax, the presence of free air in the pleural space, is the result of a rupture in the tracheobronchial tree or of a tear in the visceral or parietal pleura. The accumulated air causes the lung to collapse, effectively producing an arteriovenous shunt. The raised intrapulmonary pressure impairs venous return to the heart. The overall result of these changes is systemic arterial hypoxaemia and consequent tissue hypoxia.

There are three types of pneumothorax:

1. *Simple pneumothorax.* In the majority of cases the air leak is caused by sudden non-penetrating trauma to the chest wall which momentarily raises the intrathoracic pressure. If this occurs against a

closed glottis and a tensed diaphragm the air within the lung and airways is compressed and ruptures the pulmonary parenchyma. While road traffic accidents are the commonest cause of pneumothorax, it is not unusual for coursing Greyhounds or Whippets that fall over at speed to suffer similar damage.

2. *Open pneumothorax.* Open pneumothorax is caused by a penetrating wound of the chest wall that allows communication between the pleural space and the atmosphere. This results in a total and immediate collapse of the lung on the affected side, and air can be heard entering the chest wound with each breath. The usual causes are stake injuries or dog fights where the canine teeth penetrate the skin and tear away pieces of intercostal tissue.

3. *Tension pneumothorax.* Tension pneumothorax is the most severe form of pneumothorax, and constitutes a dire emergency. It usually results from a pleural tear acting as a one-way valve, so that air accumulates in the pleural space during inspiration but is prevented from escaping during expiration. This raises the intrapleural pressure above that of the atmosphere, and collapses the lung. It also causes the mobile mediastinum to be displaced from the midline, further collapsing the remaining functional lung. Severe hypoxaemia develops rapidly, and circulatory collapse follows almost immediately.

Pneumothorax should be suspected on clinical evidence and confirmed by radiography. Clinical signs common to all three types include:

1. Dyspnoea.
2. Muffled or absent respiratory and/or cardiac sounds.
3. Hyper-resonance of the chest.

In addition, a sucking wound, with or without subcutaneous emphysema, will be evident in animals suffering from the open type of pneumothorax because hissing can be heard. The features of a tension pneumothorax may include orthopnoea (a fixed hyperexpanded chest with reduced range of respiratory movement) and clinical signs of shock.

Radiography may be necessary to identify mild cases of simple pneumothorax, and is essential for monitoring the progress of the patient. The radiographic signs (*Fig.* 3.5) include:

1. Separation of the cardiac silhouette from the sternum in the recumbent lateral projection.
2. Absence of vascular markings at the periphery of the lung fields.

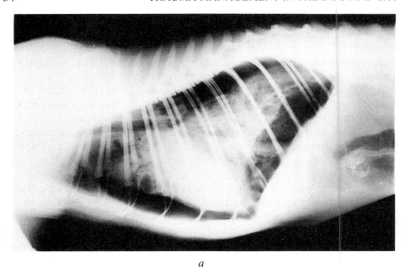

*a*

*b*

Fig. 3.5. Pneumothorax in a cat. In the lateral recumbent view (*a*) the cardiac silhouette is raised from the sternum and the lung lobes are collapsed. The dorsoventral view (*b*) shows the pneumothorax to be predominantly left-sided.

3. A widened air-filled pleural space with rounding of the costophrenic angles.

A resting animal can often tolerate a mild pneumothorax; if it is not unduly dyspnoeic when breathing room air, cage rest alone is appropriate. The air leak usually seals itself within a few hours and the free intrapleural air is resorbed over the next few days. However, the degree of dyspnoea should be monitored every few hours, and if the animal deteriorates, thoracocentesis is indicated. If air reaccumulates within 2–3 hours of thoracocentesis, the leak is generally severe enough to warrant intermittent or continuous chest drainage.

Thoracotomy may be required to repair the tear surgically if continuous suction over 48 hours fails to seal it, but fortunately this is rare. Peripheral tears in the lung can be repaired with fine absorbable suture material on an atraumatic needle using the Parker-Kerr technique developed for oversewing bowel. The tear is clamped and a continuous suture is inserted across the crushed tissue by oversewing the clamp. Alternative bites of tissue are taken either side of the clamp so that each stitch loops over the jaws. The clamp is then loosened and gently withdrawn while maintaining traction on the ends of the sutures. This inverts the crushed tissue and closes the tear. The ends of the suture are then taken through the adjacent tissue in a series of small bites so that they are easily tied together. Once the suture has been tied it is important that the lung is not overinflated for risk of tearing it again. More extensive tears are best treated by performing a lobectomy.

A tension pneumothorax must be treated by immediate thoracocentesis. It can be recognized in an emergency by inserting an intravenous catheter (or a needle if a catheter is not immediately available) with a syringe attached, into the affected hemithorax. The positive intrapleural pressure will push out the barrel of the syringe. If the dyspnoea is particularly severe, it is wise to evacuate the air initially with a catheter, three-way stopcock and syringe, using minimal restraint, until the animal's condition is less critical. Thoracocentesis using a larger drainage tube can then be performed with less risk.

## PNEUMOMEDIASTINUM AND SUBCUTANEOUS EMPHYSEMA

A less serious, although often spectacular, condition may arise from rupture of the lung tissue in the hilar region. Instead of the air entering the pleural cavity and causing a pneumothorax, it tracks along the interstitial connective tissue of the bronchial tree to the hilus, where it enters the mediastinum. The air then dissects along the mediastinum and collects in the subcutaneous tissues of the neck and face (*Fig.* 3.6). This subcutaneous emphysema may reach quite dramatic proportions, and take days or weeks to subside, but is rarely dangerous.

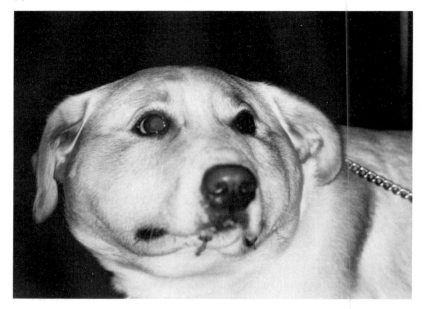

*Fig.* 3.6. A Labrador-cross with extensive subcutaneous emphysema of the face and neck. Such emphysema will usually resolve over a period of 7–10 days.

Pneumomediastinum may also occur as a result of deep wounds to the neck, tracheobronchial leaks and oesophageal ruptures. In the absence of these conditions, most cases of pneumomediastinum will resolve with cage rest and limited exercise.

If necessary, the presence of air within the mediastinum and the subcutaneous tissues can be confirmed radiographically. The presence of a pneumomediastinum is best seen on a lateral projection of the chest, when the air, acting as a negative contrast agent, provides a clear outline of the cranial mediastinal vessels and of the walls of the oesophagus and trachea (*Fig.* 3.7).

## INTERCOSTAL TEARS

Intercostal tears occur occasionally, allowing the lungs to infiltrate through the defect in the chest wall. The overlying skin remains intact so that a visible subcutaneous swelling appears with each breath. The significance of these tears depends upon the size of the defect; small tears may heal spontaneously, while large defects require surgical repair.

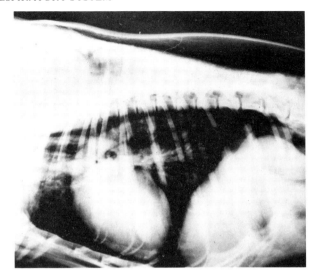

*Fig*. 3.7. Pneumomediastinum in a dog. The vessels of the cranial mediastinum are delineated by the surrounding air. Note also the subcutaneous emphysema.

## PULMONARY CONTUSION

Pulmonary contusion is caused by rapid compression–decompression forces to the chest wall or airways. This damages the capillaries and small vessels resulting in intrapulmonary haemorrhage. The alveoli are flooded with blood and adjacent small airways may become obstructed. If an extensive volume of lung is affected, hypoxaemia can be significant. Clinical signs include dyspnoea, tachypnoea, pale sometimes cyanosed mucous membranes and, occasionally, haemoptysis. Râles or areas of reduced respiratory sounds may be detected by auscultation in severe cases. The diagnosis is confirmed radiographically. Affected areas appear as patchy alveolar densities with air bronchograms, although in some cases a whole lobe (or lobes) may appear consolidated (*Fig*. 3.8).

Treatment depends upon the extent of the condition and whether there is concomitant pathology. Small contusions with no complications should be treated conservatively by restricted exercise. Broad spectrum antibiotic therapy should be employed as a prophylactic measure against pneumonia in the affected lung tissue. The trachea should be aspirated if there is a significant accumulation of blood or secretions, and in severe cases oxygen administration may be beneficial.

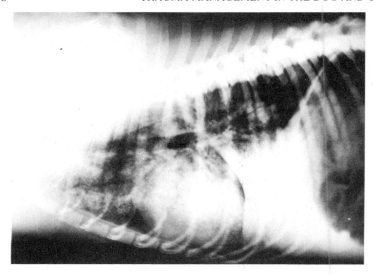

*Fig.* 3.8. Lateral thoracic radiograph showing a widespread alveolar pattern. This is typical of pulmonary haemorrhage but may also indicate pulmonary oedema or infection.

Alveolar filling may continue for several hours after the injury and it is possible to aggravate the condition by overtransfusion of the patient. As a rough estimation it is unwise to exceed $30\,\mathrm{ml\,kg^{-1}\,h^{-1}}$ of crystalloid fluid. Colloids such as plasma, blood or Haemaccel (Hoechst) are probably safer.

## PULMONARY LACERATIONS

Lacerations of the lung may result from penetrating injuries, but more commonly follow violent compression forces. There may be associated fractures of the ribs. The consequences are a pneumohaemothorax and pulmonary contusion.

The initial treatment is thoracocentesis. If the tear is minor it often seals within a few hours, but with severe damage a continuous leak of blood and air is seen. Continuous thoracocentesis over 24–48 h will encourage sealing of the defect and progress should be monitored by regular radiographic examination. A persistent leak, as evidenced by continuous drainage of blood and air, suggests a significant rupture, and in extreme cases an exploratory thoracotomy is indicated. The damaged pulmonary tissue should be treated by either a wedge resection or a lobectomy, depending upon the extent of the laceration.

## HAEMOTHORAX

Haemothorax, the accumulation of blood in the pleural space, may follow laceration of the pulmonary parenchyma or damage to any intrathoracic vessels. Its significance will depend upon the volume and the rate of the blood loss. Bleeding from the venous circulation is generally self-limiting, whereas damage to the higher pressure vessels, such as the intercostal or broncho-oesophageal arteries, is likley to be of much greater significance. At the extreme end of the scale, lacerations of the major vessels or the cardiac chambers are likely to be fatal before treatment can even be attempted.

Haemothorax has a dual significance. Pulmonary ventilation is impaired as the free pleural blood prevents lung expansion, and the animal may show signs of hypovolaemic shock due to blood loss. The pleural fluid will result in dyspnoea, tachypnoea, muffled heart and respiratory sounds and hyporesonance of the ventral chest.

The presence of pleural fluid can be confirmed radiographically, but the nature of the fluid can only be ascertained by thoracocentesis. Radiography must be performed with extreme care and the patient should not be turned on to its back.

Radiographic signs of pleural fluid (*Fig.* 3.9) include:

1. Collapse of the lung lobes.
2. A fluid density between the lung margins and the thoracic wall.
3. 'Fissuring' of the fluid between the lung lobes.

Treatment of haemothorax depends upon its severity. In mild cases thoracocentesis and cage rest will be adequate, but in severe cases the initial treatment should be rapid intravenous fluid therapy to combat the hypovolaemia. This may encourage further bleeding so that continuous thoracocentesis must be performed.

Most cases of haemothorax will respond to conservative treatment, but if severe bleeding continues, an exploratory thoracotomy should be considered.

## CARDIAC TAMPONADE

Haemorrhage into the intact pericardium will result in cardiac tamponade. This is usually caused by rupture of one of the cardiac chambers or the coronary vessels, and the increasing pressure within the pericardial sac results in reduced cardiac filling and a dramatic drop in cardiac output. The diagnosis is generally based on clinical signs which include muffling of the heart sounds, loss of the apex beat, congestion of the superficial veins and a weak, thready pulse. Confirmation of the condition can be difficult, but radiographic

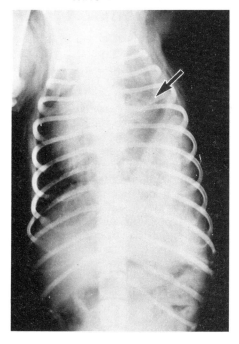

*Fig.* 3.9. Dorsoventral radiograph of a dog's thorax demonstrating unilateral pleural fluid. Note the fissure between the cranial and middle lung lobes (arrow).

evidence of pericardial fluid, demonstrated by a sharply defined globular cardiac silhouette (*Fig.* 3.10), is highly suggestive in the trauma case. In theory the pericardium can be opened and the source of the haemorrhage identified, but in practice this is rarely, if ever, attempted. In most cases, if the animal survives the initial injury, conservative treatment is the best course. The blood will be resorbed from the pericardial cavity over the next few days.

## CHYLOTHORAX

Chylothorax, the accumulation of intestinal lymph in the pleural space, is an uncommon sequel to thoracic trauma. It generally has an insidious onset, taking several days or even weeks before a clinically significant volume of fluid accumulates. As with any other pleural fluid, a definitive diagnosis can only be made following thoracocentesis. Aspiration of a milky fluid is highly suggestive, but laboratory analysis is necessary to confirm the finding.

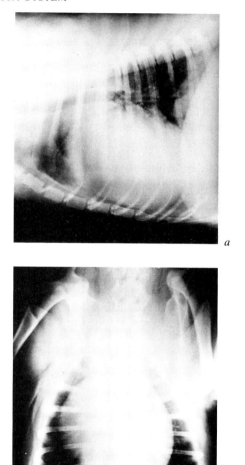

*Fig.* 3.10. Cardiac tamponade in a dog. The enlarged cardiac shadow is rounded. The dorsoventral view (*b*) emphasizes the typically sharply delineated round cardiac silhouette.

Repeated thoracocentesis (whenever the volume of chyle becomes clinically significant) combined with a low fat diet may allow the duct to seal spontaneously. If this is unsuccessful, surgical ligation of the thoracic duct is indicated, although it may be difficult to identify all the branches of the duct as it enters the chest through the diaphragm.

## PYOTHORAX

Pyothorax may develop as a result of a number of conditions but is not a common sequel to trauma. Foreign body penetration or fight injuries are possible causes, but most traumatically induced pyothoraces follow a perforating injury to the oesophagus. In many cases the perforation is due to the sharp edges of a piece of bone lacerating the oesophageal wall. The leakage of food and saliva provokes an intense mediastinitis and pleural effusion soon follows. Dysphagia, dyspnoea and ptyalism should indicate the likely cause of injury, and the diagnosis is confirmed by oesophagoscopy and radiography. Radiographic signs include a pneumomediastinum or a widened mediastinum with a fluid density and evidence of pleural fluid. Contrast radiography using a non-ionic water-soluble iodine compound such as iohexol (Omnipaque, Nyegaard) may be useful in confirming an oesophageal rupture. The non-ionic compounds do not provoke a mediastinitis such as is seen with barium sulphate when they leak into the perioesophageal tissues.

Surgical repair is necessary since it is most unlikely that the oesophagus will heal spontaneously. Adequate exposure is attained using a lateral thoracotomy. The oesophageal mucous membrane is closed with an everting continuous horizontal mattress suture, and its muscular coat coapted with simple interrupted sutures.

## RUPTURED DIAPHRAGM

Diaphragmatic rupture is a common sequel to blunt thoracic trauma. The severity of the condition depends on the site and extent of the tear and effects range from sudden death due to massive lung collapse or rupture of a major vessel, to less severe cases where lung volume is reduced by a lobe(s) of the liver, the stomach or the intestines entering the chest. Dyspnoea may be aggravated by changes in posture or by feeding. In the case of a left-sided rupture the stomach almost invariably enters the chest, so that a gastric dilatation or torsion is always a potential hazard. In the right-sided rupture the liver generally enters the chest and is often accompanied by a partial torsion of the posterior vena cava. Thoracic transudate is thus a common additional finding, and causes further reduction in functional lung volume.

The diagnosis is based upon clinical findings and confirmed radiographically. Solid viscera within the chest may result in muffled or displaced heart sounds and a displaced apex beat. Intestinal borborygmi may be heard and percussion may reveal hyporesonance in the vicinity of solid viscera, or hyper-resonance over trapped loops of bowel or stomach.

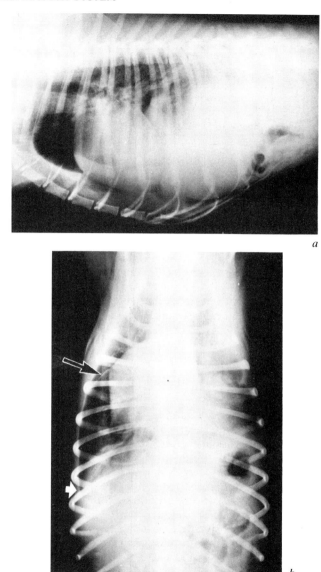

*Fig.* 3.11. *a*, Lateral view of a dog's thorax. The diaphragm cannot be seen clearly and there is evidence of pleural fluid. *b*, The interlobar fissure (black arrow) and rounding of the costophrenic angle (white arrow) suggest there is also fluid in the right hemithorax. The fundic gas shadow is displaced cranially. Diagnosis: diaphragmatic rupture with pleural fluid.

Common radiographic signs associated with diaphragmatic rupture (*Fig*. 3.11) include:

1. Loss of the diaphragmatic line.
2. Abdominal organs within the thorax displacing the thoracic structures.
3. Gas-filled loops of bowel within the thorax.
4. The presence of pleural fluid.
5. Cranial displacement of the fundic shadow in cases of left-sided rupture.

In doubtful cases the position of the stomach and small intestines can be verified by contrast radiography using 8–12 ml/kg (100 per cent wt/vol) barium sulphate suspension (*Fig*. 3.12).

The diaphragmatic rupture must be repaired surgically. A gas-filled distended stomach or an incarcerated abdominal organ demands immediate surgery, but in general anaesthesia can be delayed until the animal's condition is stable.

A ventral midline laparotomy provides good access to both sides of the chest and enables inspection of the abdominal viscera for other evidence of damage. It may be necessary to enlarge the tear before repairing it in order that the trapped viscera can be returned safely to the abdomen. Particular care should be taken that the posterior vena cava is not occluded when the liver is manipulated. The possible presence of adhesions should be borne in mind, but they rarely present a significant surgical problem.

Postoperative drainage of the surgical pneumothorax is essential. It is not sufficient to hold the lungs in full expansion while the last suture is tied. The repaired diaphragmatic rupture is unlikely to be airtight, and while the laparotomy wound is being closed air will enter the chest. Even after closure, the pneumoperitoneum may be slowly sucked through the diaphragmatic defect, and many animals die following an apparently adequate repair because the surgical pneumothorax is not eliminated.

Development of pulmonary oedema is not uncommon postoperatively. This generally follows overinflation of lung tissue that has been collapsed for a long period of time. It is particularly important that the lungs are not over-zealously re-expanded in such cases. It is far safer to encourage re-expansion by gentle thoracocentesis after the chest has been closed.

Successful repair calls for close cooperation between the surgeon and the anaesthetist. Induction of anaesthesia may precipitate a cardiac arrest, particularly in the hypoxaemic animal, and it is important that the surgeon rapidly opens the abdomen and relieves the pressure on the lungs. It is a wise precaution for the surgeon to scrub for surgery prior to induction of anaesthesia and to be prepared to act quickly.

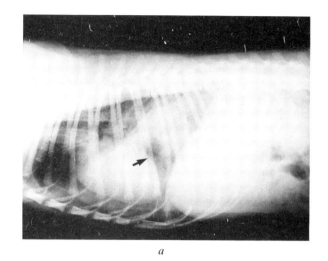

*a*

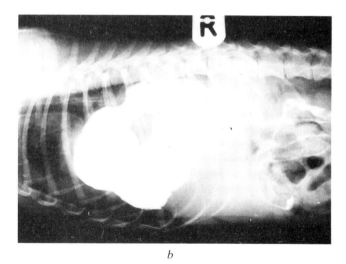

*b*

*Fig.* 3.12. *a*, Lateral radiograph of a dog's chest with displacement of the cardiac silhouette, an abnormal gas shadow in the chest (arrow) and a soft tissue line running from the heart base. Diagnosis: suspected diaphragmatic rupture. *b*, Lateral radiograph of the same dog after administration of barium sulphate by mouth. The stomach is almost entirely within the chest, confirming the diagnosis of diaphragmatic rupture.

Chapter 4

# *The Abdomen*

Damage to abdominal viscera should always be considered a possible sequel to any traumatic accident and may be divided into closed and open injuries.

### Closed abdominal injury

Closed abdominal injuries are far less common in dogs and cats than in man, probably owing to the relatively high inertia of the human body compared to that of the smaller animals. The symptoms of closed abdominal injury are rarely obvious and are slow to develop, so it is important that the animal's condition is assessed over a series of examinations.

Abdominal pain is always present but it is difficult to differentiate between pain arising from peritoneal irritation and that from muscular damage to the abdominal wall. Blood loss in the post-traumatic period is life-threatening, and if the patient has suffered multiple injuries, such loss may be difficult to assess. Blood lost into the thoracic cavity may be easily demonstrated by radiography, and significant haemorrhage into limb muscles may be obvious from local swelling. However, if the patient develops a rapid and fading pulse, with marked pallor of the mucous membranes, and no other signs of haemorrhage, it is highly likely that blood has been lost into the abdominal cavity. Abdominal radiography may be useful, but the signs are variable, depending on the volume of free fluid and its position. A uniform density throughout the abdominal cavity, which obscures gas-filled bowel loops and masks the borders of solid viscera, is suggestive of free fluid. It is best seen in the recumbent lateral projection. Paracentesis may help to confirm suspicion of abdominal haemorrhage, but, under these circumstances, there should be no hesitation in performing an exploratory laparotomy. If there is no abdominal catastrophe, then little harm will be done, but, if bleeding points in the abdomen can be located, haemorrhage can be controlled and the animal's life saved. When an exploratory laparotomy is performed in these circumstances it is essential that this is done through an incision of adequate size. Bleeding vessels and other signs of soft tissue damage are difficult to find in an abdominal cavity which is already full of blood, and this is made doubly difficult if the exploration is carried out through a keyhole incision.

Symptoms from damaged viscera or from injuries to the urinary system may be delayed for hours or even days. Unexplained vomiting is often the earliest sign of developing peritonitis due to intestinal leakage, and the first indication of bladder rupture may be that the patient has not passed urine (assuming that it is adequately hydrated).

Rupture of the body wall may occur when the intra-abdominal pressure rises suddenly as a result of a crushing accident. The cat is particularly prone to this injury, and the muscles generally tear around the costal or pelvic margins. The viscera may be palpated subcutaneously, and the defect in the body wall is usually obvious. Repair is generally straightforward, and the defect is closed with horizontal mattress sutures. On rare occasions the body wall is pulled away from the pubis leaving little tissue to which the body wall can be sutured. In this case it may be necessary to use stainless steel sutures taken through a number of holes drilled in the anterior aspect of the pubis.

### Open abdominal injury

Open wounds of the abdomen are generally obvious but the hair should be clipped to allow a thorough inspection. It is important to remember that the size of the surface wound may bear little or no relation to the extent of the injury to the underlying structures and all such wounds must be thoroughly explored. For example, the skin wound caused by an airgun pellet is quite small, but is often accompanied by multiple puncture wounds of the bowel and solid viscera.

The abdominal organs most likely to be damaged by direct trauma are the solid viscera (liver, spleen and kidney), the gastrointestinal tract and the distal urinary system. The hepatic biliary system, the pancreas and the ureters, by virtue of their anatomical position and relative mobility, are less likely to be injured.

### THE LIVER

Rupture of the liver may cause profound haemorrhage, and animals with a history of trauma and signs of abdominal pain, intra-abdominal haemorrhage and hypovolaemic shock require aggressive therapy. Radiography may demonstrate free fluid in the abdomen, but paracentesis is of more value since it will identify the fluid. Intravenous fluid administration should be started immediately, and the animal prepared for exploratory laparotomy.

Liver tissue is soft and friable and does not offer a good basis for suturing. Massive liver disruption may prove impossible to treat, but bleeding from even quite considerable superficial tears may often be controlled by suturing. The basic technique is to use fine absorbable sutures on a large curved atraumatic needle. These are inserted deep into the liver tissue or sometimes completely through the full thickness of the lobe. They are then tied tightly enough to arrest bleeding but not so tight as to cut the liver as though with a cheese wire. The sutures should be inserted at least 1 cm from the edge of the tear, and ideally should interlock in order to provide continuous pressure along the surface of the tear (*Fig.* 4.1). Sometimes the bleeding may be partially controlled by incorporating surgical absorbable sponge into the edges of the tear before inserting the sutures.

Severe damage to a liver lobe may necessitate a lobectomy or at least a partial lobectomy of the affected portion. Partial lobectomy is

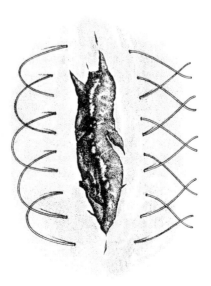

*Fig.* 4.1. Interlocking horizontal mattress sutures will help to control bleeding from the cut surface of the liver.

performed by bluntly separating the liver tissue and ligating each major vessel. Mattress sutures are preplaced in the free edge of the tissue that is to be retained before the vessels are ligated. A similar technique is employed to remove an entire lobe; in this case the vessels are ligated at the hilus.

## EXTRAHEPATIC BILIARY SYSTEM

Rupture of the gallbladder or bile ducts is often associated with hepatic trauma. In these circumstances the abdominal fluid may develop a green tinge, but free blood generally masks the bile. The extrahepatic biliary system should always be checked for signs of damage when the liver is repaired. Alternatively, if hepatic damage is minor, and the rupture is overlooked, accumulation of free bile in the abdomen will result in a chemical peritonitis. Its severity and course will vary with the rate at which the bile is leaking. Slow accumulation may initially result in rather vague signs, and the cause of the peritonitis does not become apparent until the patient becomes jaundiced.

The ruptured ends of the common bile duct may be anastomosed over a short polypropylene catheter but the surgical procedure is not easy and leakage is always a potential hazard. If there is any doubt as to the viability of the repair it is preferable to anastomose the gallbladder to the antimesenteric border of the distal duodenum with a two-layer inverting side-to-side technique. Rupture of one of the divisional ducts is not a major problem since bile from the affected lobe will drain through the remaining duct system following ligation of the torn ends. Rupture of the gallbladder itself is most easily managed by removal of either the damaged portion or the whole organ.

## THE SPLEEN

Splenic rupture may be due to straightforward trauma or to rupture of tumours, such as haemangiomas and haemangiosarcomas. Tears in the spleen may be dealt with using a similar technique to those described for the liver, but if splenic damage is extensive, then splenectomy is the safest course. If bleeding is severe, it is wise to clamp all the splenic vessels with artery forceps before applying individual ligatures.

## THE PANCREAS

Blunt trauma to the pancreas may cause release of digestive enzymes and result in fat necrosis and peritonitis. Partial pancreatectomy is generally required, although minor tears can be repaired by suturing the pancreatic capsule. Careful sharp dissection between the lobes is preferable to cutting across them, and the exposed area should be oversewn with a continuous suture in the capsule. Since chromic catgut is subject to enzymic digestion non-absorbable sutures such as silk should be used.

## INTESTINAL DAMAGE

Unexplained vomiting following trauma is often the earliest sign of a developing peritonitis. Abdominal guarding may not be an obvious sign, but the patient is clearly ill and shows the classical signs of water and electrolyte depletion. Diagnosis of peritonitis can be confirmed radiographically by the presence of ill defined pockets of intra-abdominal gas, but it should be appreciated that such changes are not always obvious (*Fig.* 4.2).

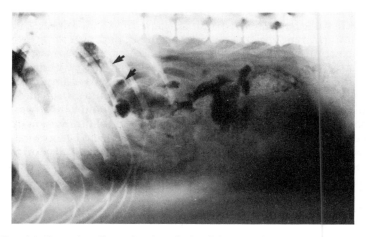

*Fig.* 4.2. Lateral radiograph of a dog's abdomen with peritonitis and a pneumoperitoneum. The abdomen has a granular appearance and the wall of the colon (arrows) is unusually obvious as it is outlined by intra- and extraluminal gas.

Damage to the gut may arise from tearing of the mesenteric blood supply, from bruising and ultimate sloughing of the intestinal wall, or from actual disruption of the intestinal tract.

Damage to the mesentery with extensive haematoma formation is not in itself an indication for excision provided that the adjacent intestine has an adequate blood supply. If there is ischaemia of a length of bowel this must be resected back to a point where the vascular supply is adequate. Tears in the mesentery should be closed in order to avoid a subsequent volvulus. Disruption of the bowel or extensive bruising necessitate débridement of the damaged bowel ends and anastomosis. Tears involving the upper part of the duodenum may prove difficult to anastomose because the mesoduodenum is short. It may be necessary to oversew the end of the duodenum and perform an end-to-side anastomosis with the adjacent jejunum.

When intestinal contents have leaked into the peritoneal cavity it is essential that adequate peritoneal lavage is carried out, using isotonic saline at body temperature. It is important to remember that peritoneal reaction to intestinal contents will continue for a time after the stimulus is removed, and it is important to maintain adequate fluid therapy for at least 48 hours after the operation. Small amounts of water and soft food can be offered 24 hours after surgery.

## THE KIDNEYS

Intra-abdominal haemorrhage and anterior abdominal pain are usually seen following renal trauma, and an exploratory laparotomy may be required to establish whether the bleeding is renal, splenic or hepatic.

Blood loss resulting from massive renal damage can be sufficiently severe to cause death or profound hypovolaemic shock within minutes. In less severe injuries haemorrhage from the kidney may be subcapsular, retroperitoneal or within the peritoneal cavity, depending upon whether the capsule is lacerated and the position of the tear. Subcapsular haematomas are rarely associated with specific clinical signs and are resorbed without additional treatment. If the tear does not involve the peritoneum, the haematoma will be retroperitoneal and may be large enough to be palpated.

Radiography may confirm suspicion of renal damage, but contrast techniques are often required to evaluate the injury fully. Plain radiographs will reveal gross changes in kidney outline and size, and may suggest retroperitoneal haemorrhage. However, excretory urography best determines the site and extent of the damage. A 'low volume, high dose' technique (see Chapter 8) should be used since the uptake of the contrast material is dependent upon renal function. Restricted renal perfusion and/or parenchymal damage will reduce the uptake and result in poor filling of the collecting system.

Tears in the kidney parenchyma may be closed by inserting a continuous absorbable suture in the tough renal capsule, but if necessary the sutures may penetrate quite deeply into the renal cortical tissue. Haemorrhage from the kidney may be temporarily controlled by isolating the renal artery and applying a tape ligature or a bulldog clamp for a short period. It is inadvisable to use Spencer Wells forceps as these may produce permanent damage to the arterial wall.

In cases where gross renal damage has occurred, it may be safest to remove the whole kidney and its ureter.

## THE URETERS

Ureteral rupture is an uncommon sequel to abdominal trauma. Urine usually spills into the abdomen, but if the outflow from the kidney is obstructed, hydronephrosis will develop. Treatment depends upon the site of the rupture, the extent of the damage, and renal function. Excretory urography will identify the site of the rupture and enable kidney function to be evaluated; plain radiography is rarely helpful.

Anastomosis of the ureter is technically difficult and it may be advisable to remove both the ureter and associated kidney. Careful examination of the other kidney is essential before a nephrectomy is considered.

Ruptures of the distal end of the ureter may be treated by anastomosing the ureter to the proximal part of the bladder. The ureter should be pulled through a prepared subserosal tunnel before it is sutured to the bladder mucosa. The length of the tunnel should be at least three times the diameter of the ureter. This tunnel acts as a valve and prevents reflux of urine into the ureter from the bladder.

## THE BLADDER

Rupture of the bladder and spillage of urine into the peritoneal cavity often passes unrecognized and it is essential that any accident case is carefully observed to ascertain whether there is an adequate urine output. Rupture of the bladder may be diagnosed by a variety of methods; the simplest is to insert a urinary catheter and then introduce a quantity of air. Subsequent radiographs will show a normal pneumocystogram if the bladder is intact, otherwise air will be dissipated throughout the peritoneal cavity. As an alternative, retrograde urography using a water-soluble iodine compound may be used. If the bladder is ruptured, the contrast agent will leak through the tear and can be seen free in the abdomen (*Fig.* 4.3).

---

*Fig.* 4.3. (*opposite*) *a*, Lateral abdominal radiograph of a German Shepherd dog. There is loss of detail in the ventral abdomen and the bladder cannot be seen. *b*, The same dog following intravenous urography. The outlines of one kidney and both ureters can be seen. The bladder outline is irregular and free contrast material can be seen in the abdomen (arrows). Diagnosis: rupture of the bladder. *c*, The same dog following introduction of further contrast material into the bladder by retrograde urography. The intra-abdominal contrast is more obvious.

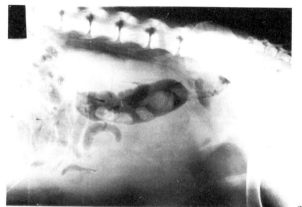

*a*

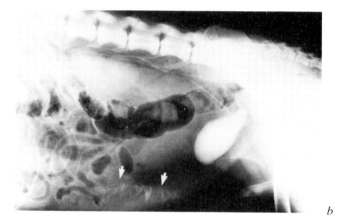

*b*

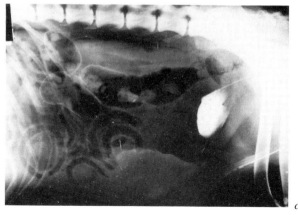

*c*

Repair of a ruptured bladder is usually straightforward and the bladder wall is closed in two layers. However, when the tear extends into the urethra the repair is technically more difficult. In some cases repair is not possible and it may be necessary to close as much of the bladder as possible and then to insert a Foley catheter into the bladder. The catheter is left in place for 7–10 days during which time the urethra and bladder neck will heal. In the male dog it is necessary to insert the Foley catheter through a high urethrostomy.

In the majority of cases urine in the abdomen evokes only a slight reaction. None the less, it is advisable to irrigate the peritoneum with isotonic saline before the abdomen is closed. Following surgical repair of the bladder it is particularly important to ensure that the animal can urinate spontaneously. If no urine is passed within 8 hours of surgery the bladder should be carefully catheterized and, if necessary, gently irrigated.

In cases where a catheter is left in the bladder it is essential that patency of the catheter is checked regularly since its end may become blocked by a blood clot. This may lead to gross dilatation of the bladder and possible breakdown of the repair. The patency of an indwelling catheter may easily be checked by injecting 5 ml of sterile water or saline up the catheter. This will also remove any obstructing material.

Chapter 5

# *The Nervous System*

The brain and spinal cord are soft, friable structures which are particularly sensitive to external trauma. They are supported and protected partly by the meninges and CSF and partly by the bony cranium and the vertebrae. However, as the brain is totally enclosed by this rigid cranium, any increase in brain volume will result in an increase in intracranial pressure and is a potential cause of brain damage.

The pathological changes that follow trauma to the brain can be classified as concussion, contusion and laceration. Concussion is the mildest type of injury and is generally defined as unconsciousness following trauma in the absence of any permanent physical damage. Intraparenchymal haemorrhage and cerebral oedema are seen with contusion. Lacerations, the most severe type of injury, are generally associated with considerable disruption of the normal architecture of the brain.

Haematomas are classified as epidural or subdural. Epidural haematomas generally result from a cranial fracture rupturing the middle meningeal artery; this causes a rapidly expanding mass to form between the skull and the dura. Subdural haematomas occur as a result of a rupture of the small vessels that are found in the pia mater and similarly cause pressure on the underlying brain tissue.

Injuries to the spinal cord are generally associated with vertebral column damage, although concussion of the spinal cord in the absence of bony damage may occur occasionally. Vertebral fractures or luxations may sever the cord but more commonly cause cord compression. Traumatic disc protrusions generally produce an impact type of injury, and the subsequent oedema and swelling may exert additional pressure on the cord.

55

Central nervous system trauma is always challenging to diagnose and treat. The lesion must be located and the extent of the damage assessed. Prognosis can sometimes be given early, but generally the patient's condition must be monitored over several hours or even days before the eventual outcome can be predicted.

Neurological examination should be preceded by the usual physical examination and any life-threatening conditions such as hypoxia, haemorrhage and shock treated immediately. Hypoxia is a common complication of head injuries and aggravates cerebral oedema. Maintenance of a patent airway and adequate ventilation must take priority over all other procedures. Shock is not commonly seen in animals suffering from CNS injury alone. Neurological examination should be performed before analgesics or sedatives are given so that the patient's responses are not affected. Opiate analgesics raise intracranial pressure and they should not be used in animals with a head injury.

## TRAUMA TO THE BRAIN

It may be difficult to perform a complete neurological examination in a patient suffering major head injuries, since the animal may be incapable of reacting to stimuli. This makes assessment of postural reactions and spinal cord reflexes impossible and may also make it difficult to interpret other tests. The following are generally the most useful signs in assessment of head injuries:

1. Level of consciousness.
2. Pupil size and reaction.
3. Posture and motor function.
4. Altered vital signs.

These should be monitored regularly so that any deterioration in the animal's condition can be treated.

### Level of consciousness

A number of altered mental states can be recognized, these include:

(*a*) decreased awareness (recognition of owner, perception of painful stimuli such as toe pinching);
(*b*) stupor, coma;
(*c*) convulsions.

Although stupor and coma are superficially similar, it is possible to rouse the stuporous animal by stimulating it vigorously. The comatose animal, however, is unable to respond to any external stimuli. Most cases of post-traumatic coma in dogs are due to haemorrhage into the midbrain and brain stem. The coma is often transient, lasting only a few minutes, followed by a rapid recovery. In such cases the prognosis is generally favourable. However, when coma persists for several hours it indicates severe brain injury and a poor prognosis.

Convulsions following head injuries are generally due to haemorrhage, cerebral oedema or depressed cranial fractures.

Haemorrhage often produces a space-occupying subdural or epidural haematoma and a consequent increase in intracranial pressure. Management of these cases includes a craniotomy.

### Pupil size and reaction

It is important to assess whether abnormal ocular reflexes are due to injuries of the nervous system or of the eye itself. An ophthalmic examination should be performed, and both fundus and anterior chamber examined. Retinal haemorrhage or detachment will result in abnormal pupillary responses which may mimic those seen in brain damage.

Both the direct and consensual pupillary responses should be assessed. Pupils which are bilaterally constricted, bilaterally dilated or asymmetrical suggest damage to the midbrain. Horner's syndrome due to damage to the cervical sympathetic trunk also results in asymmetric pupils. Asymmetric or bilaterally constricted pupils carry a better prognosis than those that are bilaterally dilated. Pupils that progress from constriction to dilatation indicate deterioration in the patient's condition, but a change from abnormal to normal pupil size is a good prognostic sign.

### Posture and motor function

Common signs relating to dysfunction of the vestibular system include:

(a) head tilt;
(b) spontaneous nystagmus;
(c) abnormal gait.

Abnormal motor responses may also be manifested as:

(a) decerebrate rigidity;
(b) decerebellate rigidity.

Vestibular dysfunction following head injuries is generally central in origin but the possibility of peripheral vestibular disease must be

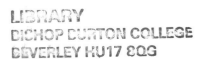

eliminated. Peripheral vestibular dysfunction involves the inner and middle ear, and may be due to a fracture of the petrous temporal bone. The external auditory canal should be checked for signs of haemorrhage, which often occurs in association with this fracture.

Head tilt is seen with both types of vestibular dysfunction. The lesion is on the same side as the ear that is directed towards the ground.

Spontaneous nystagmus may also be associated with both types of dysfunction. Spontaneous nystagmus due to brain stem injury may be horizontal, vertical or rotary. Vertical nystagmus is not seen in peripheral disease. The fast phase of the horizontal or rotary nystagmus is directed away from the side of the lesion. Animals with bilateral vestibular defects may not exhibit head tilt or nystagmus, but their head movements are usually exaggerated.

Gait abnormalities should be assessed if the animal's condition permits. The animal may circle towards the side of the lesion and often prefers to walk alongside a solid object such as a wall. In severe cases the animal may be unable to stand and will merely roll over and over. Circling and rolling can be seen in both peripheral and central dysfunction but leaning is associated with the peripheral form alone. Leaning occurs towards the side of the lesion and is due to an imbalance between the flexor and extensor tone of the trunk muscles. It should be distinguished from hemiparesis where there is obvious muscle weakness of one side.

Ataxia, especially if severe, and unilateral hypermetria may indicate damage to the brain stem or cerebellum, but following trauma, the majority of ataxic patients have spinal cord lesions.

The neurological signs of vestibular dysfunction are summarized in *Table* 5.1.

*Table 5.1.* **Neurological signs of vestibular dysfunction**

|                        | Central                        | Peripheral           |
| ---------------------- | ------------------------------ | -------------------- |
| Head tilt              | +                              | +                    |
| Spontaneous nystagmus  | Horizontal, vertical or rotary | Horizontal or rotary |
| Circling or rolling    | +                              | +                    |
| Leaning                | −                              | +                    |
| Ataxia                 | Severe                         | Mild                 |
| Hemiparesis            | +                              | −                    |
| Hypermetria            | +                              | −                    |

Decerebrate and decerebellate rigidity both result in quadrilateral extensor rigidity and opisthotonus. However, in decerebrate rigidity there is complete extensor rigidity while in decerebellate rigidity there is alternating flexion and extension of the hindlimbs. The presence of other signs of cerebellar dysfunction, such as head tremor and nystagmus, helps to distinguish between decerebrate and decerebellate rigidity.

Animals with decerebellate rigidity have a more favourable prognosis than those with decerebrate rigidity, and it is important to distinguish between the two types. If decerebellate rigidity progresses to decerebrate rigidity the prognosis is extremely poor.

### Altered vital signs

Regular monitoring of the animal's temperature, pulse and respiration provides useful information about the progress of the patient. Single estimations are of relatively little value and the general pattern of changes should be assessed. Increased intracerebral pressure will at first result in slowing of the pulse and respiratory rates and a rise in body temperature. Later, as the effects of hypoxia become evident, the pulse will become weak and rapid, breathing will be shallow and fast, and body temperature will continue to rise.

Although monitoring vital signs may be useful in assessing the extent of the brain injury, the integrity of specific cranial nerve reflexes may also help to localize the lesion. Cranial nerve dysfunction that appears to be spreading to involve adjacent nerves suggests the cranial lesion is expanding and indicates a worsening prognosis.

Depending upon the condition of the animal, the cranial nerves can be assessed as in *Table* 5.2.

## TREATMENT OF HEAD INJURIES

Initial management of head injuries should aim to prevent or control cerebral oedema and haemorrhage. Treatment may have to be modified in the light of the patient's progress, and surgery may be required if the animal's condition deteriorates despite therapy.

Cerebral oedema should be treated with relatively high doses of intravenous dexamethasone (1–4 mg/kg every 4–8 h). This is probably safer than infusing hypertonic mannitol. Mannitol used as a 20 per cent solution (at 2 g/kg) is an osmotic diuretic and is most effective in reducing cerebral oedema. However, it should not be used where intracranial haemorrhage is suspected. Mannitol reduces cerebral oedema and thus the size of the brain. This increases the potential space for epidural or subdural haemorrhage. Mannitol may also leak into the brain parenchyma through damaged capillaries. Later, when plasma osmolarity is restored, fluid from the extracellular space is drawn into the nervous tissue, inducing further cerebral oedema. It is safer to use mannitol when there is a breach in the cranium, as in cranial fractures or during surgery, since there is room for expansion.

*Table 5.2. Assessment of cranial nerves*

| Cranial nerve | Signs of dysfunction | Test |
|---|---|---|
| II | Visual impairment | Visual placing test |
| | | Menace reaction |
| | Unequal pupil size | Eyes following movement of light or cottonwool ⎫ with III |
| | Dilated pupils | Pupillary reflexes ⎭ |
| III | Dilated pupils | *See* II |
| | Ptosis | |
| | Ventrolateral strabismus | |
| IV | Dorsomedial strabismus | |
| V | Loss of jaw tone | Maxillary/ophthalmic reflex ⎫ |
| | | Palpebral reflex ⎬ with VII |
| | | Corneal reflex ⎭ |
| VI | Medial strabismus | Horizontal eye movement when following objects |
| VII | Paralysis of facial muscles of expression | *See* II and V |
| VIII | Deafness | Handclap |
| | Nystagmus | |
| | Headtilt | Righting reflexes |
| | Loss of balance | |
| IX | Dysphagia | Gag reflex with X |
| X | Dysphagia | *See* IX |
| | | Laryngeal reflex |
| XII | | Tongue retraction |

Cerebral hypoxia must be avoided at all costs, and if necessary the animal must be intubated and given oxygen. IPPV may be required in some cases.

Intravenous fluid therapy may be required. This will depend on any other injuries present and the length of time the animal is unable to take fluids by mouth. Overtransfusion must be avoided because of the risk of inducing or aggravating cerebral oedema. Measurement of urinary output and central venous pressure will give some indication of the state of the circulation.

**Surgical treatment**

Surgery is indicated when the patient's condition deteriorates despite medical treatment. Radiography of the skull may help to indicate the extent of cranial fractures, but the films are often confusing. Taking several different views of the cranium will help to 'skyline' the bony lesion (*Fig.* 5.1), and the two sides should be examined for asymmetry. However, regular and frequent assessment of the patient is generally of more value in deciding whether surgery is required.

Before surgery begins, an attempt should be made to decide whether the deteriorating neurological signs are due to brain stem haemorrhage or to extracerebral pressure. Extracerebral pressure may be due to cerebral oedema, subdural or epidural haematomas and depressed fractures. These carry a reasonable prognosis after decompressive surgery. In contrast, the prognosis for brain stem haemorrhage is extremely poor.

Uncorrected extracerebral pressure will result in tentorial herniation in which the cerebral hemispheres are forced under the tentorium cerebelli and the midbrain is compressed (*Fig.* 5.2). This in turn results in brain stem haemorrhage so that the neurological signs of advanced tentorial herniation are similar to primary brain haemorrhage. The two conditions can be distinguished by their different time scales; signs of primary brain stem haemorrhage develop immediately after trauma, whereas the signs of tentorial herniation may take hours or even days to develop (*see Table* 5.3).

Cases that require surgery fall into two categories. The first contains all those requiring emergency decompressive surgery. These generally show the following:

1. Deteriorating level of consciousness.
2. Signs of advancing tentorial herniation (pupillary responses particularly relevant).
3. Deterioration of vital signs (pulse and respiration in particular).

The second group contains those cases with depressed cranial fractures whose neurological state is stable. This includes animals with:

1. Fractures depressed more than the thickness of the skull.
2. Fractures where fragments are embedded in the brain.
3. Open fractures.

Surgery is relatively straightforward in the second group of patients, and the temporalis muscle provides reasonable protection for the brain in the postoperative period. Management of the first group is more demanding, however, and should, if possible, be referred to a specialist centre if there are insufficient resources available for such exacting surgery and postoperative care.

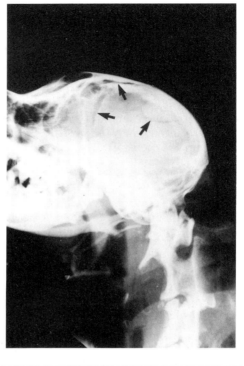

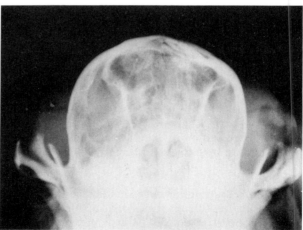

*Fig.* 5.1. *a*, Lateral radiograph of a dog's skull showing multiple fracture lines (arrows). *b*, Rostro-caudal view of the same skull to skyline the fracture. Note the depressed fragment.

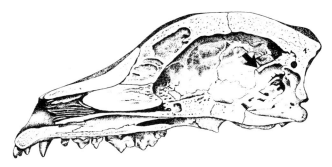

*Fig.* 5.2. Tentorial herniation. The cerebral hemispheres may be forced under the tentorium cerebelli (arrow) with increased intracranial pressure.

*Table 5.3.* **Comparison of acute brain stem haemorrhage with tentorial herniation following head injury**

|  | *Brain stem haemorrhage* | *Tentorial herniation* |
|---|---|---|
| Onset | Early | Delayed |
| Course | Static to progressive | Progressive |
| Pupils | Constricted early, dilated late | Unilateral dilatation, progresses to bilateral dilatation |
| Consciousness | Stuporous to comatose | Alert or apathetic progressing to coma |
| Muscle tone | Decerebrate rigidity or flaccid paralysis | Normal or weak progressing to flaccid paralysis |
| Reflexes | Usually symmetrical | Often unilateral asymmetry |

Reproduced with permission from Oliver J.E. (1972) Neurologic emergencies in small animals. *Vet. Clin. North Am. [Small Anim. Pract.]* **2**, no. 2, 344.

Elevation of depressed cranial fractures is best performed through a flap incision in the skin. The temporalis muscle is reflected and any free bone fragments carefully removed. Major fragments can be wired in position, but it is generally quicker and safer to remove them completely. Fragments which are still attached are carefully elevated. The temporalis muscle is sutured along its attachment before the skin is closed.

## SPINAL CORD TRAUMA

Traumatic injuries of the spinal cord are often the result of vertebral column damage. Vertebral fractures, luxations or subluxations and protrusion of an intervertebral disc are the most commonly seen.

Radiography is generally of more value in assessing damage to the spine than in the investigation of head injuries. However, radiography only provides information as to the position of the vertebrae *at the time of the radiographic examination*. The only radiographic sign of a spontaneously reduced luxation may be a slightly misplaced vertebra or a narrowed disc space, but the damage to the cord is often considerable.

Spinal cord injuries can be classified as concussion, compression or various degrees of transection.

### Cord concussion

This is due to local pressure changes around a limited section of the spinal cord. Radiographic evidence of vertebral canal damage is rarely seen, and the effect varies from mild impairment of nervous conduction to complete failure.

### Cord compression

Cord compression is often the result of crushing fractures of the vertebral body or of epiphyseal fractures in immature dogs. These injuries usually cause acute local pain with protective muscle spasm.

### Cord transection

Cord transection may be complete or incomplete, and is often the result of fractures, luxations and subluxations. Radiographic examination will demonstrate the site of any *skeletal* injury and demonstrate the type and extent of the damage to the vertebral column (*Fig.* 5.3). A neurological examination will indicate the severity and the position of the *cord* injury.

Animals with damage to the vertebral column must be moved extremely carefully in order to avoid further damage to the cord. When possible, a board or tray should be placed underneath the patient, but in any case the animal must be carefully supported when it is moved.

Neurological examination should be as thorough as possible, but the spine should not be manipulated excessively. This is particularly important when cervical fractures are suspected.

### Neurological examination

The objective of a neurological examination is to assess whether the spinal cord damage is of upper motor neurone (UMN) or lower motor neurone (LMN) origin (*Fig.* 5.4), and to determine the level of the

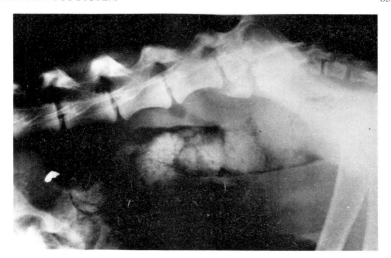

*Fig.* 5.3. Lateral radiograph of a Bloodhound's spine with a displaced fracture of the seventh lumbar vertebra. Radiography will demonstrate the site and extent of the skeletal damage but provides little information regarding the neurological injury.

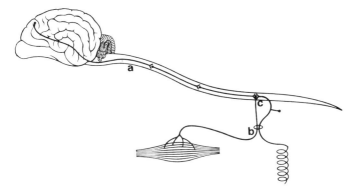

*Fig.* 5.4. Upper motor neurone injuries are generally due to damage to the corticospinal tract within the spinal cord (a). Lower motor neurone injuries involve the peripheral nerve (b) or the nerve outflow from the cord (c).

damage. Examination must establish (*a*) the state of the cord below the injury and (*b*) whether there is any conduction across the injured area.

Injuries to cord segments involving the brachial outflow (C6–T2) and the lumbar outflow (L4–S1) are LMN type and have dramatic

*Table 5.4.* **Checklist for neurological examination**

Posture:

| Forelimbs | L | R | Hindlimbs | L | R |
|---|---|---|---|---|---|
| paralysis/paresis | | | paralysis/paresis | | |
| proprioception | | | proprioception | | |
| muscle tone | | | muscle tone | | |
| limb withdrawal | | | limb withdrawal | | |
| pain perception | | | pain perception | | |
| triceps reflex | | | crossed extensor reflex | | |
| | | | Perineal reflex | | |
| | | | Panniculus response | | |

effects on the fore and hindlimbs. Paralysis or paresis, loss of tone and loss of local reflexes are seen. It may be difficult, however, to interpret loss of function in a fractured limb. There may be peripheral nerve damage, as in radial paralysis associated with a humeral fracture, but it is more likely that the fracture is preventing the limb from being used. Similarly it is important to differentiate between loss of function due to pain and that due to a neurological lesion.

The corticospinal system can be damaged anywhere between the cerebral cortex and the LMN, but the majority of UMN injuries are due to damage to the cord. These are characterized by reduced voluntary movement, intact or hyperactive reflexes, increased tone and the presence of abnormal reflexes. It cannot be assumed that the cord rostral to the innervation of a limb is undamaged simply because limb reflexes are present. Paraplegic animals with complete transection of the thoracic cord may still make rhythmical stepping movements with the hindlimbs if the tail or hindquarters are stimulated by pinching. They may also be able to wag their tails if the perineum is stimulated.

It is advisable to follow a set plan and to tabulate the findings of the examination. This aids interpretation and provides a checklist (*see Table* 5.4). The animal's posture should be noted first. Decerebrate and decerebellate rigidity have already been described and should be differentiated from the Schiff–Sherrington syndrome which may be seen when the spinal cord is transected between T2 and L4 (as in fracture luxations of the lower thoracic region). The syndrome is characterized by rigid extended hypertonic forelimbs and flaccid hypotonic hindlimbs. The spinal reflexes are intact and forelimb sensation and voluntary motor function are normal.

Proprioception should be assessed in each limb if the patient's condition permits. The limb is displaced either by placing the foot on a sheet of paper which is then slowly pulled out so that the leg is

abducted, or by flexing the carpus or extending the hock and resting the leg on the dorsum of the paw. Inability to return the displaced limb to its normal position is one of the earliest signs of cord damage.

The panniculus response can be used to establish the level of the cord injury. The sensory component of the reflex is segmental from T1 to L3 while the motor fibres are derived only from C8 to T2. If the arc is intact, pricking the skin of the dorsal trunk generates impulses which travel via the ascending fibres within the cord to produce a reflex skin twitch. Since the afferent fibres of the reflex are arranged in segments it is generally possible to determine the level of cord damage. The skin is pricked on both sides of the midline, starting just in front of the ilium and slowly moving forwards until a twitch is provoked. If the cord lesion is not extensive, it may be possible to establish not only the level of the injury but also whether the lesion is bilateral or unilateral.

The integrity of the reflex arcs distal to the cord injury may be assessed by testing local reflexes such as the patellar and triceps reflexes and the pedal withdrawal response.

Conduction across the injured area of cord can be assessed by examining the animal's response to a painful stimulus. This can be done when the pedal withdrawal response is investigated. The web of the foot of the toe is stimulated by applying a pair of artery forceps or by a vigorous pinch. Limb withdrawal merely indicates that the reflex is intact. However, if the animal appears to feel pain, this confirms that afferent impulses are able to travel across the section of injured cord to the brain. Such conscious perception of pain, demonstrated by the animal crying out, attempting to bite or turning to look at the foot, is a favourable sign.

A crossed extensor reflex indicates an UMN injury since it is an abnormal reflex associated with severe cord damage. Flexion of one hindlimb elicits extension of the other, and is seen when hindlimb withdrawal reflexes are tested.

Most lesions of the spinal cord will cause altered function caudal to the lesion. *Table* 5.5 summarizes the type of damage that can be expected from complete cord transection at various different levels.

The prognosis for an animal with spinal cord trauma depends upon both the extent of the injury and whether the damage is reversible. It can be difficult to forecast the outcome, but the presence or absence of pain perception is probably the most significant sign. Absence of pain perception indicates a grave prognosis. *Table* 5.6 summarizes how the severity of cord damage may be correlated with the neurological signs.

**Radiological examination**

The spine should be radiographed after the neurological examination. The whole spine should be examined in case multiple injuries are

Table 5.5. *Effect of complete cord transection at levels indicated*

| Segment | Forelimb reflexes | Hindlimb reflexes | Perineal reflexes |
|---------|-------------------|-------------------|-------------------|
| C1–C4   | UMN               | UMN               | UMN               |
| C5–T2   | LMN               | UMN               | UMN               |
| T2–L4   | Unaffected        | UMN               | UMN               |
| L4–S1   | Unaffected        | LMN               | UMN               |
| S1–S3   | Unaffected        | Unaffected        | LMN               |

UMN injury characterized by
  reduced voluntary movement
  hyperactive spinal reflexes
  increased tone
  abnormal spinal reflexes

LMN injury characterized by
  paralysis
  loss of spinal reflexes
  reduced tone

Table 5.6. *Estimation of spinal cord damage severity using neurological signs*

| | Degree of cord damage | | |
| Sign | Mild | Moderate | Severe |
|------|------|----------|--------|
| Paralysis | +/− | + | + |
| Loss of pain perception | − | − | + |
| Crossed extensor reflex | − | − | + |
| Loss of bladder control | − | +/− | + |
| Schiff–Sherrington syndrome | − | − | +/− |

+, present; −, absent.

present. For example, a LMN injury of the brachial outflow will mask a UMN injury of the upper cervical region and if only the lower cervical spine is radiographed the second injury may be missed.

Extreme care in positioning the animal is essential. Undue struggling must be avoided to prevent further injury, and general anaesthesia is usually required to obtain diagnostic films. The spine should not be manipulated excessively during anaesthesia as loss of protective muscle spasm makes it easier to damage the cord inadvertently when there is a vertebral fracture or luxation.

The animal must be carefully positioned to avoid false narrowing of the intervertebral spaces, and the spine should be packed with radiolucent foam wedges, as shown in *Fig.* 5.5. Lateral and ventrodor-

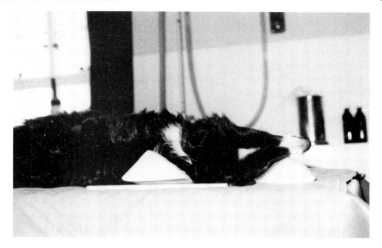

*Fig.* 5.5. Foam wedges are used as radiolucent padding to ensure the spine is parallel to the radiographic plate.

sal views should be taken as luxations may be missed on a lateral view (*Fig.* 5.6). Coning down on to a small area of the spine will improve radiographic detail and is particularly valuable when minor changes are suspected.

Myelography is rarely necessary to localize the site of cord compression in the traumatized patient. It may be indicated in those cases that are suitable candidates for decompressive surgery where the exact level of the cord injury is unclear. However, the information gained from plain radiographs, combined with clinical findings, is generally adequate.

## TREATMENT OF SPINAL CORD TRAUMA

The aim of treatment is to reduce pressure on the spinal cord and to provide good nursing care that will encourage the animal's recovery. Treatment may be conservative or surgical, but if surgery is to be successful it must take place within a few hours.

### Surgical treatment

Surgery is indicated for the following:

1. Decompression of the cord in a paralysed animal.

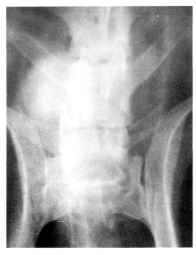

*a*

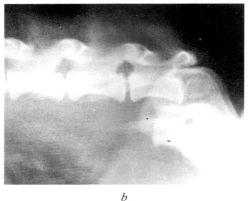

*b*

*Fig.* 5.6. *a*, Ventrodorsal view of the lumbar spine. There is a fracture-luxation of L6/7. *b*, Lateral view of the same injury. It is important to take radiographs of the spine in at least two planes in order to assess the full extent of the damage.

2. Immobilization of significantly unstable vertebrae.

Animals that are able to perceive pain distal to the injury are better candidates for surgery than those that cannot. It is doubtful whether surgery is justified in a paraplegic animal that cannot perceive pain, unless it is performed within 6 hours of the onset of signs.

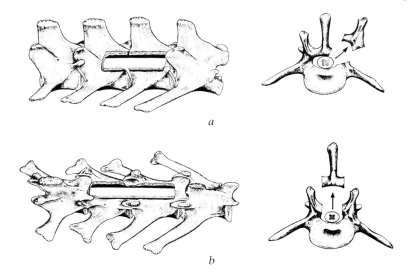

*Fig.* 5.7. *a*, Hemilaminectomy; *b*, dorsal laminectomy.

Decompression can be achieved either by hemilaminectomy or dorsal laminectomy (*Fig.* 5.7). However, since laminectomy involves removal of the dorsal spines it is impractical if these are required for internal fixation to immobilize a fracture.

The decision to operate and immobilize an unstable vertebra will be influenced by the radiological findings. Compression fractures are generally stable and do not require internal fixation whereas unstable fractures should be immobilized. The greater the vertebral instability the greater the likelihood of callus formation as the fracture heals. This callus may compress the cord and produce significant neurological deterioration several weeks after the initial injury.

Immobilization is usually achieved by stabilizing three or four dorsal spines on either side of the fracture. Spinal plates or bolts may be used, or alternatively a stainless steel pin can be bent around the spines and wired to them (*Fig.* 5.8).

### Medical treatment

Animals with minor vertebral injuries and insignificant neurological deficits are suitable candidates for medical treatment. These include cases with stable fractures or minimally displaced subluxations where voluntary movement and pain perception is still present. Dexamethasone (2 mg/kg) should be given intravenously twice daily for the first

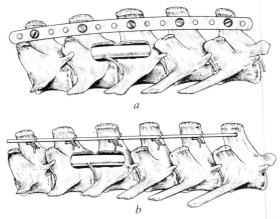

*Fig.* 5.8. Vertebral fractures may be repaired with (*a*) spinal plates, (*b*) a pin and wire.

24–48 hours to reduce the initial oedema and inflammation of the spinal cord. Anti-inflammatory therapy can then be continued with oral prednisolone (1 mg/kg) or betamethasone (0·1 mg/kg) for a further 5–7 days.

Rest is an essential part of conservative treatment. Hospitalization and cage rest is usually far more successful than trying to manage the animal at home. High quality nursing is essential, and particular attention must be paid to the comfort of the patient. Animals with neurological deficits are particularly prone to pressure sores. Clean dry bedding, careful washing, drying and regular turning all contribute to the patient's well-being, and liberal use of non-perfumed talc will help to reduce pressure sores.

Animals with a paralysed bladder require extra nursing care. A LMN injury to the sacral nerves or a more proximal UMN injury will both cause bladder paralysis. Flaccid paralysis is seen in LMN injury, while in UMN injury, because the reflex arc is still intact, reflex emptying may occur.

If the bladder is allowed to become overdistended the detrusor muscle will lose its tone and dribbling overflow will result. This may cause irreversible damage to the detrusor muscle so that when reflex emptying returns it is no longer effective. Inadequate bladder emptying may also lead to retention cystitis and secondary bacterial infection of the urinary tract. Overdistension is best avoided by keeping the bladder catheterized. The cat's bladder can usually be expressed manually, but undue force should not be used so that the bladder wall is not damaged. Even so, a catheter is more satisfactory, since bladder emptying is more complete. Many animals with a poor micturition reflex, but which are able to feel pain distal to the injury, recover the use of their bladder if overdistension and cystitis can be avoided.

Chapter 6

# The Musculoskeletal System, the Skin and the Eye

## THE MUSCULOSKELETAL SYSTEM

Initial management of fractures and joint injuries should prevent any further damage to the affected limb and minimize the development of complications during repair. Conditions such as delayed or non-union healing of fractures, infection and impaired articular function can be prevented with good initial care.

Road traffic accidents and jumping from heights are the commonest causes of musculoskeletal injuries. Less frequently they are the result of crushing injuries, shooting, kicks and blows. A wide variety of musculoskeletal pathology is seen but it is rarely a threat to life. However, concomitant thoracic, abdominal or neurological injuries are common, and these must be treated first. Hypovolaemic shock rarely results from uncomplicated musculoskeletal trauma and is generally associated with injuries to other organs.

Whenever there are injuries of the proximal forelimbs, chest radiographs should be taken in order to detect any thoracic damage not already revealed by the clinical examination. Without this, pulmonary haemorrhage and pneumothorax can easily be overlooked, and, if untreated, may prove disastrous if the animal has to be anaesthetized. Similarly, when there are fractures of the pelvis or upper hindlimb, the possibility of rupture of the urinary bladder must be considered if it cannot be palpated. Urethral patency should also be checked in these circumstances, by catheterization if necessary.

A detailed examination of the injured limb should be delayed until the animal's general condition is stable. Bony, articular and soft tissue damage, including any skin wounds, should then be assessed. These injuries should be handled sympathetically since they will be painful.

73

Palpation of the foot and distal limb will indicate the temperature of the extremity and provide valuable information about its vascular supply. An area that is colder than the corresponding area of the other side suggests that peripheral circulation may be compromised. This may result in devitalized tissue that will eventually slough. This is more likely where there is gross soft tissue damage such as in gunshot injuries than in closed fractures. Devitalized skin which subsequently sloughs may convert a closed fracture into an open one.

Peripheral oedema commonly develops after long bone fractures as a result of impaired venous and lymphatic drainage as well as from the inflammatory reaction. It usually resolves over a few days once the fracture is immobilized, but its initial development should be limited by bandaging. Oedema is easily recognized as a swelling that 'pits' when pressed with a finger.

Peripheral nerve damage should be assessed during the detailed examination. Knowledge of the sensory and motor distribution of the peripheral nerves enables an accurate assessment of their condition to be made (*Fig.* 6.1). Pinching the skin with a haemostat and noting the animal's response is generally sufficient, although some stoic patients may not react even when sensation is normal.

Peripheral nerve injuries are classified according to their severity. Neuropraxia is usually the result of nerve contusion and occurs after minor stretch injuries. There is generally no permanent damage, and function returns within a few days. Axonal degeneration occurs after the more severe axonotemesis which is a sequel to severe stretch injuries (such as occurs in brachial plexus avulsions). Recovery depends on regrowth of the nerve distal to the injury and proceeds at approximately 1 mm per day. Fibrosis at the damaged site may impair or prevent nerve regeneration. Neurotemesis is a consequence of complete disruption of the nerve and is generally associated with open wounds. Fortunately this is not a common complication of limb trauma.

A fracture which communicates with the outside via a breach in the skin is termed an open fracture. These are classified according to the extent of the tissue damage. First degree open fractures have little soft tissue damage and the wound is the result of a sharp fragment of bone puncturing the skin. Second degree fractures have more extensive soft tissue damage due to perforation from the outside. There is usually considerable contamination of the wound and underlying tissues. Third degree fractures have extensive bone and soft tissue damage. Gross contamination is seen such as occurs in crushing injuries or when the animal has been dragged along the road.

Closed fractures are less likely to become infected, nevertheless further damage to the surrounding tissues must be avoided. It is particularly important that a closed fracture is not converted into an open fracture by careless handling of the patient.

Joint injuries are a less frequent result of trauma than fractures, but luxations and fracture-luxations are not uncommon. They are more common in the adult animal, as a similar force applied to the young animal tends to fracture the adjacent growth plate.

Diagnosis of fractures and luxations is based on the clinical findings and is confirmed by radiography. The clinical signs of both injuries include deformity, swelling, pain, crepitation and loss of function. Radiographs should always be taken in two planes. Undisplaced or minimally displaced fractures and certain luxations can easily be overlooked if one view only is taken (*Fig.* 6.2).

Initial management of all musculoskeletal injuries should include adequate analgesia. Opiates are the drugs of choice, but it should be emphasized that immobilization of the injured part will also help considerably to reduce the pain.

## Closed fractures

Fractures distal to the elbow and stifle can be immobilized using splints, casts or Robert Jones bandages. Aluminium Zimmer splints are satisfactory for small dogs and cats, but are not strong enough to immobilize fractures in large dogs. Commercially available foam padded plastic splints are useful in these cases, and can be broken along prescored lines to fit the limb. All splints should be applied over a well-padded bandage, and the ends must not protrude beyond the end of the padding. Too much padding can be counter-productive and may result in pressure sores if it becomes compressed and rucked up. This is most likely to occur in long term use when the animal is weight bearing and is not a major problem when external fixation is used as a temporary measure.

The splint must immobilize the joints proximal and distal to the fracture. A splint that ends close to a fracture can be detrimental as it may actually increase movement at the fracture site.

A bulky conforming bandage such as the Robert Jones is particularly effective for immobilization of fractured limbs as it provides firm but gentle support. It is applied using rolls of absorbent cotton wool which is then compressed with conforming bandages and elasticated tape. Pressure is evenly distributed and the soft tissues are protected. The success of this type of dressing depends upon the use of sufficient padding. Some 2–3 kg of cotton wool are required for a 20–25 kg dog.

Initially a stirrup is applied to the dorsal and ventral surfaces of the foot in order to attach the bandage to the limb (*Fig.* 6.3). The cotton wool is then wrapped around the leg and compressed with conforming bandages. The stirrup is turned back on itself so that it is incorporated into the layers of conforming bandage (*Fig.* 6.4). The bandage is

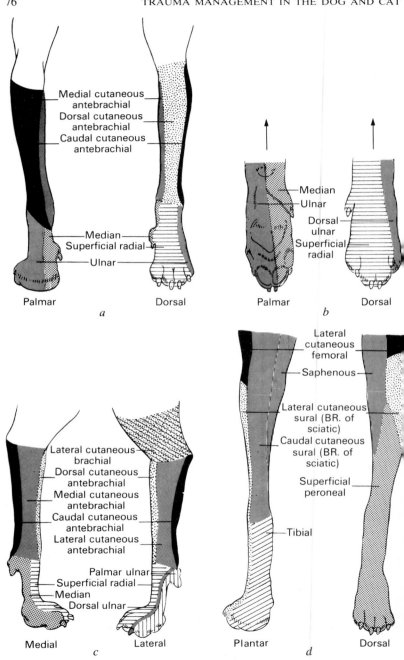

Medial cutaneous
antebrachial
Dorsal cutaneous
antebrachial
Caudal cutaneous
antebrachial

Median
Superficial radial
Ulnar

Palmar                        Dorsal
*a*

Median
Ulnar
Dorsal
ulnar
Superficial
radial

Palmar                        Dorsal
*b*

Lateral cutaneous
brachial
Dorsal cutaneous
antebrachial
Medial cutaneous
antebrachial
Caudal cutaneous
antebrachial
Lateral cutaneous
antebrachial

Palmar ulnar
Superficial radial
Median
Dorsal ulnar

Medial                        Lateral
*c*

Lateral
cutaneous
femoral
Saphenous

Lateral cutaneous
sural (BR. of
sciatic)
Caudal cutaneous
sural (BR. of
sciatic)

Superficial
peroneal

Tibial

Plantar                       Dorsal
*d*

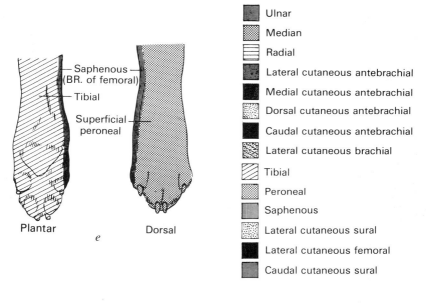

| | Ulnar |
| | Median |
| | Radial |
| | Lateral cutaneous antebrachial |
| | Medial cutaneous antebrachial |
| | Dorsal cutaneous antebrachial |
| | Caudal cutaneous antebrachial |
| | Lateral cutaneous brachial |
| | Tibial |
| | Peroneal |
| | Saphenous |
| | Lateral cutaneous sural |
| | Lateral cutaneous femoral |
| | Caudal cutaneous sural |

Saphenous (BR. of femoral)

Tibial

Superficial peroneal

Plantar        Dorsal

*e*

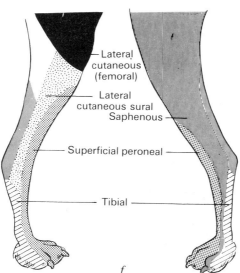

Lateral cutaneous (femoral)

Lateral cutaneous sural

Saphenous

Superficial peroneal

Tibial

*f*

*Fig.* 6.1.  Areas innervated by the peripheral nerves of the fore (*a–c*) and hind (*d–f*) limbs. (Reproduced with permission from: Hoerlein B. F. (1978) *Canine Neurology: Diagnosis and Treatment.* Philadelphia, Saunders.)

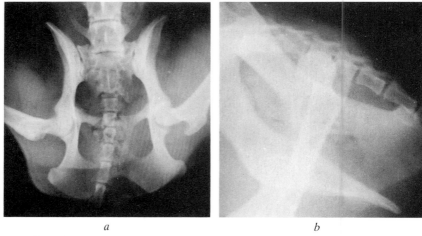

*Fig.* 6.2. Radiograph of a luxated hip: ventrodorsal view (*a*), oblique view (*b*). The luxation may be overlooked if only a single view is taken.

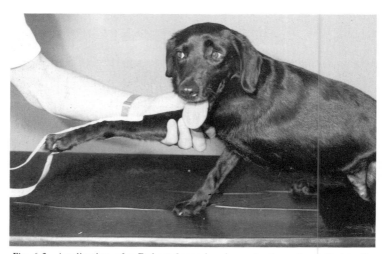

*Fig.* 6.3. Application of a Robert Jones bandage. A stirrup is applied to the dorsal and ventral aspects of the foot before cotton wool is wrapped around the limb. The tape should not encircle the limb lest it impede circulation to the foot.

further compressed by wrapping elasticated tape around the whole dressing (*Fig.* 6.5).

Fractures above the elbow and stifle are much less suitable for external support, and cage rest is usually the only alternative. The relatively large muscle masses surrounding the humerus and femur act

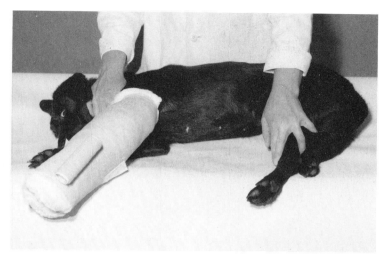

*Fig.* 6.4. The stirrup is turned back and incorporated between the layers of conforming bandage. This will prevent the bandage from slipping.

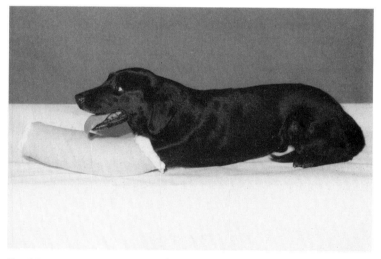

*Fig.* 6.5. The bandage is completed using elasticated tape. This type of bulky conforming bandage provides good support for injured limbs.

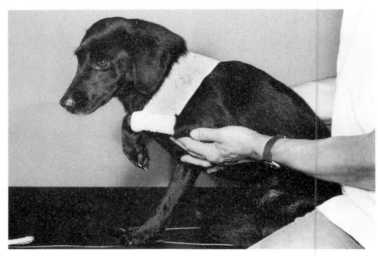

*Fig.* 6.6 Application of a Velpeau sling. The bandage is taken around the forearm and the chest.

as natural splints, and further support is often unnecessary. Where support is required for the shoulder a Velpeau sling is effective. A length of bandage holds the flexed forelimb close to the chest so that the foot is unable to slip out anteriorly and the elbow cannot move posteriorly. A bandage is used to wrap the forearm and is then taken over the shoulder and round the chest (*Fig.* 6.6). It is then taken behind the elbow of the opposite limb and continued over the carpus of the flexed leg (*Fig.* 6.7). The bandage is taken round the chest a second time and brought over the flexed elbow before it encircles the chest a third time and finishes by covering the carpus again (*Fig.* 6.8). The bandage is then taped to itself to prevent the elbow and carpus from slipping out.

If internal fixation is likely to be required antibiotic therapy should be started at the time of initial treatment. A broad spectrum bactericidal agent such as ampicillin or a potentiated sulphonamide should be given parenterally so that adequate circulating blood concentration is achieved prior to surgery.

**Open fractures**

In contrast to closed fractures, wound sepsis is more likely to develop in the presence of an open fracture. Devitalized tissue, blood clots, foreign material such as soil and grit, and any bacteria present will all influence the extent of the problem.

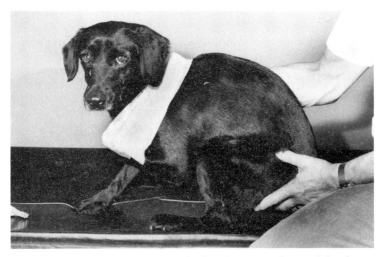

*Fig.* 6.7. The bandage is taken over the flexed carpus and around the chest a second time.

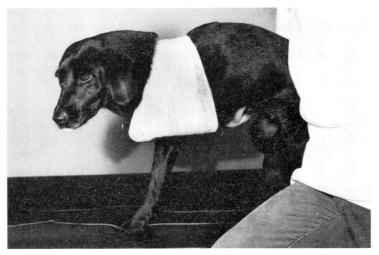

*Fig.* 6.8. The bandage immobilizes the elbow before encirling the chest again. The sling is finished by covering the carpus. The bandage should be taped to itself to prevent the elbow and carpus from slipping out.

Initial treatment should minimize further soft tissue damage. The wound should be gently flushed with sterile saline and any gross debris wiped away. The area should then be protected by a sterile non-stick dressing before any external support is applied. The dressing should be left in place until the animal's condition is stable when full treatment can be provided. In this way further contamination is avoided. Haemorrhage is usually adequately controlled by this procedure and it is rarely necessary to ligate vessels at the time of the accident. Analgesics will be required to provide adequate pain relief, and a broad spectrum bactericidal antibiotic should be given parenterally. Adequate concentrations at the site of the wound are best achieved by intravenous injection of the antibiotic as a bolus.

When the animal's condition is stable the wound can be cleaned thoroughly and the limb prepared for surgery. The hair should be clipped from a wide area around the wound with electric clippers. To prevent contamination with hair, the wound should be packed with saline-soaked swabs or water-soluble jelly (K–Y Jelly (Johnson & Johnson)). After clipping, the swabs can be removed or the jelly washed away.

Irrigation of the wound is an essential part of subsequent treatment. Large volumes of sterile water or saline are effective. Chlorhexidine (0·5–1·0 per cent) can be added to improve antimicrobial activity. Cytotoxic soaps and detergents should not be used and there is some doubt as to the efficacy of povidone-iodine solutions. Antibiotics that are unsuitable for parenteral administration, such as gentamicin or polymyxin, can be added to the irrigating solution. This may be particularly valuable in the severely contaminated wound.

The irrigant should be infused under pressure in order to improve the mechanical flushing effect. A large syringe (35 or 60 ml) or a giving set attached to an 18 gauge needle are quite adequate. Wounds where the dirt is ground in, such as occurs when the distal limb is dragged along the road, are particularly difficult to clean. Patient irrigation is required since the area should not be scrubbed or the dirt will simply be rubbed in further.

Débridement of all devitalized tissue and foreign material should be performed next. Assessing tissue viability can be difficult. The presence or absence of bleeding from a cut surface is a useful guide. A skin flap with a sharp demarcation line between normal skin and dark congested skin is less likely to be viable than one where there is a gradual transition between normal and abnormal tissue. Fat undergoes necrosis readily and should be generously excised.

Muscle should be débrided until the remaining tissue has a normal colour and consistency. Small pieces of tissue that are isolated from their blood supply should be removed, and skin edges should be cleanly excised. Damaged ligaments and tendons must be preserved.

Small pieces of bone which cannot be incorporated into the fracture repair can be discarded, but larger fragments should be washed and retained. Fragments with a periosteal attachment are particularly valuable and should be treated with special care.

Primary closure of the wound should only be undertaken at this stage if subsequent healing is assured. In doubtful cases it may be better to wait and allow the wound to granulate or to suture it 3–6 days later (delayed primary wound closure). In general first degree wounds can be sutured immediately whereas second and third degree wounds should be closed by delayed primary closure. Healing is not significantly delayed if the wound is closed by delayed primary closure. It is usually successful if débridement is adequate and if there is not undue tension on the sutures.

The optimum time for fracture repair depends on a number of factors, such as the condition of the animal, the type of fracture and the risk of infection. Each case must be judged on its own merits. First degree fractures can often be treated as closed fractures provided débridement is adequate. If internal fixation is selected, the fracture site should be exposed, if possible, through a new incision and not through the débrided area.

Second degree fractures require rigid immobilization in order to promote healing in the presence of infection. In general this is best achieved with internal fixation. The use of intramedullary pins may be counter-productive since they may introduce infection deeper into the medullary cavity and do not provide as much stability as plates and screws. Movement at such a fracture site may encourage the development of osteomyelitis.

Grade three long bone fractures are often associated with extensive loss of soft tissue and are best treated with a Kirschner–Ehmer system (*Fig.* 6.9). This uses externally clamped transcortical pins to immobilize the fracture while permitting access to the soft tissue wounds. The pins may be placed a considerable distance from the fracture site so that the risk of spreading the infection is reduced. Alternatively, the fracture can be immobilized with plates and screws, but, in this case, it is absolutely essential that complete stability is assured. If this is not achieved a non-union fracture is likely to result and the metallic implants will act as foci of infection.

Grossly contaminated wounds should be swabbed for bacterial culture when they are débrided. The type of organisms present, and their antibiotic sensitivity, can be established. In the more severe injuries antibiotic cover may be required for several weeks, and it is helpful to know which drugs are likely to be most effective.

Partial amputation of a distal extremity, loss of the tail and 'degloving' injuries are relatively common in the cat. Haemorrhage may be a significant problem and a temporary tourniquet, a pressure

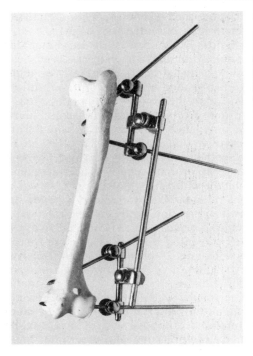

*Fig.* 6.9. A Kirschner–Ehmer splint. The outer two transcortical pins should be inserted first. The connecting bars are then loosely assembled before the inner two pins are inserted. The splint is then adjusted and tightened.

pad or ligation of blood vessels may be required before full surgical repair is performed. In all other respects these injuries should be treated as outlined above.

## Joints

Joint luxations are less common than limb fractures and are generally closed injuries. Shearing injuries of the carpus and tarsus, where part of the joint is ground away, are exceptions.

Radiographs of the joint should always be taken in two planes if a luxation is suspected. This will confirm the direction of the displacement and reveal associated fractures. This type of fracture generally requires internal fixation to provide joint stability, and is often best repaired with a tension band technique or lag screws. Radiographs will also reveal any dysplastic changes. These will result in impaired stability when the luxation is reduced and must be taken into account in the subsequent management of the case.

Closed reduction of simple luxations can be attempted as soon as the animal's general condition permits. General anaesthesia is essential, and neuromuscular blockade with IPPV can be helpful in difficult cases in dogs. Suxamethonium (0·3 mg/kg) given intravenously during anaesthesia provides 15–20 minutes relaxation. IPPV must be continued until spontaneous respiration returns once the drug is metabolized. Reversal is not required with this muscle relaxant.

Post-reduction radiographs should be taken to confirm joint alignment. 'Reluxation' is often due to unconfirmed failure of the initial attempt at replacement.

When closed reduction fails, or the joint genuinely reluxates, surgical intervention is indicated. Open reduction, with or without some form of internal stabilization, generally offers a good prognosis provided the joint is not dysplastic.

### Shoulder

Luxation of the shoulder joint is relatively uncommon. The humeral head usually luxates medially, although occasionally it may be displaced laterally. Both luxations are easily reduced by appropriate pressure on the distal scapula and proximal humerus. Postoperatively the limb should be immobilized in a Velpeau sling for 7–10 days.

### Elbow

The elbow joint invariably luxates with the radius and ulna lateral to the humerus. Luxation occurs when the joint is flexed more than 45°, thus allowing the anconeal process to be forced out of the olecranon fossa. Reduction is performed with the joint similarly flexed. The anconeal process is engaged on the lateral humeral condyle and the reduction completed by slowly extending the limb while rotating the carpus inwards and pressing on the lateral aspect of the olecranon. The limb should be bandaged for 7–10 days after reduction so that the periarticular structures may heal.

### Hip

Hip luxations are the commonest traumatic luxation in dogs and cats and the head of the femur generally moves anterodorsal to the acetabulum. Posterodorsal and ventral luxations are much less common. In order to reduce the luxation, the anaesthetized animal is placed on a table in lateral recumbency with the affected leg uppermost. A tape or small rope, suitably padded, is placed through

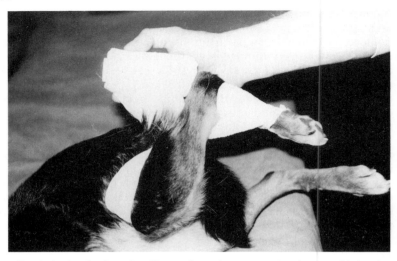

*Fig.* 6.10. Application of an Ehmer sling. The metatarsal region is padded and a figure-of-eight bandage applied around the flexed stifle and hock. The hock is rotated outwards to maintain inward rotation of the hip.

the groin and tied to the table. For an anterodorsal luxation the stifle is rotated outwards and the hip extended so that the femoral head is pulled caudally on to the rim of the acetabulum. The stifle is then rotated inwards while traction on the foot is maintained. Once the luxation has been reduced the joint should be manipulated by flexing and extending it several times, to expel any blood clots, organizing granulation tissue and remnants of torn joint capsule from the acetabulum. Moderate pressure on the greater trochanter should be applied with a palm of the hand while the hip is manipulated.

Following reduction, the hip should be immobilized in an Ehmer sling for 4–5 days to maintain flexion. The sling should also maintain abduction and inward rotation of the hip. The bandage is started by encircling the metatarsal region and continued proximally in a figure of eight around the flexed stifle so that the hock is rotated outwards and the stifle inwards (*Fig.* 6.10). A little padding below the hock will help to prevent the distal limb from swelling but too much will make the bandage slip. In short-legged dogs and those with a lot of loose skin the bandage can be taken over the back to encircle the abdomen to provide more stability.

### Stifle

Traumatic stifle luxations are relatively uncommon and are associated with severe damage to the ligaments and periarticular structures.

Generally, both cruciates and one collateral ligament are ruptured, with or without meniscal damage. The limb should be supported in a Robert Jones bandage until open reduction and surgical repair is undertaken. Closed reduction is totally unsatisfactory, since it is impossible to maintain joint stability and degenerative joint disease is inevitable.

### Hock

Hock luxations may be simple, accompanied by malleolar fractures, or occur as a result of shearing injuries with loss of periarticular structures. Simple luxations can be treated by closed reduction. The limb should be supported in a bandage for 2–3 weeks. Malleolar fractures should be repaired with a tension band wire or a lag screw. Shearing injuries are best treated initially with external support. Once soft tissue healing is under way, and infection controlled, the damaged collateral ligament should be replaced with a prosthesis.

## THE SKIN

Skin wounds must be treated on their own merits, but the same principles of irrigation, débridement and suturing apply as described in the management of open fractures. The aim of treatment is to restore the integrity of the skin with as little deformation and scarring as possible, and to minimize the amount of granulation tissue that is required to fill the defect.

It is beyond the scope of this book to describe the many techniques employed in repairing large skin defects. These are time-consuming procedures and grafting is often necessary. However, the quality of the initial wound management will have considerable influence on the final outcome. Strict maintenance of asepsis throughout treatment is essential. This is particularly important in the treatment of burns, where quite extensive areas of damaged tissue are particularly susceptible to infection.

## THE EYE

### Prolapse of the eyeball

Prolapse of the eyeball is seen most commonly in the small brachycephalic breeds that have been picked up by the scruff of the neck. This may occur in a dog fight or even after inadvertent handling. It is sometimes seen in other dogs and in cats as a result of head trauma sustained in a road traffic accident.

The prolapse must be treated as an emergency. The optic nerve is damaged and blindness is a common sequel, even if the eyeball is replaced almost immediately. Rapid treatment may not prevent the loss of sight but it will prevent further damage and desiccation of the eye itself. It is a distressing condition for the animal (and the owner) and deserves prompt treatment on these grounds alone.

The prolapsed eyeball becomes trapped outside the closed lids. It may be possible to replace it by holding the eyelids open and pressing the eyeball back into the orbit with a sterile swab moistened with saline. If this is impossible the animal must be anaesthetized and a lateral canthotomy performed. Once the eyeball has been replaced the lids should be sutured together to maintain it in position for a week while the underlying tissues heal and oedema subsides. The eyeball is likely to reprolapse if this is not carried out. In the Pekinese it may be more satisfactory to suture the third eyelid to the bulbar conjunctiva as sutures in the lids have a tendency to pull through. Systemic steroids and antibiotic cover should be provided to reduce oedema and prevent infection. Topical atropine should be used if there are signs of uveitis. Additional damage to the eyeball should also be treated. Desiccation and ulceration is most satisfactorily treated with antibiotic ointment. Repair of a ruptured cornea is outlined below.

### Eyelid wounds

Lacerations of the eyelid can cause severe deformity and consequent malfunction if they are left to granulate. The principles of repairing these wounds are as for any skin wound, but particular attention must be paid to achieving good alignment and restoring the natural shape of the eyelid. This is particularly important in lacerations that are at right-angles to the lid. Those that run parallel to the lid are less likely to gape and cause permanent disfigurement.

### Conjunctival injuries

These often appear dramatic when there is conjunctival haemorrhage, particularly where this extends into the sclera as well. However, it is rarely necessary to provide more than antibiotic cover for complete resolution.

### Intraocular haemorrhage

Blood that has accumulated in the eye without penetration of the cornea should be left to resolve without surgical interference. Occasionally glaucoma develops because drainage through the filtration angle is blocked with blood. In this case paracentesis should be performed to remove as much blood as possible and to reduce intraocular pressure. Treatment with carbonic anhydrase inhibitors and miotics may be required later if the glaucoma persists. If there is associated iritis, atropine should be applied topically into the eye, two to three times daily. The atropine, by producing pupillary dilatation, should prevent the development of adhesions between the iris and other parts of the anterior chamber. Atropine should not be used if there is evidence of glaucoma.

### Corneal injuries

Superficial corneal injuries heal rapidly and require only antibiotic cover. These injuries are painful and analgesic therapy with opiates or non-steroidal anti-inflammatory drugs is unlikely to delay healing and will certainly improve the animal's well-being. It may be necessary to use topical local anaesthesia to examine the eye thoroughly and to remove any foreign bodies.

Penetrating corneal injuries must be repaired, under general anaesthesia, as soon as possible after injury in order to provide the best chance of recovery of normal function and to minimize permanent scarring. The repair is easier to perform if it is carried out before severe corneal oedema develops, usually within a few hours of injury.

The anterior chamber is cleared of blood and any foreign material by flushing with sterile normal saline. If the iris is prolapsed it is replaced as nearly as possible into its normal position. The corneal defect is sutured with 6/0 polyglactin 910 (Vicryl, Ethicon) or polyglycolic acid (Dexon, Davis and Geck). The anterior chamber can be re-expanded with an injection of sterile saline. Antibiotic cover should be provided with ophthalmic ointment or subconjunctival injection. Chloramphenicol is the antibiotic of choice and can also be given systemically as it is the only antibiotic which crosses the blood–aqueous barrier. Topical aureomycin has also been used successfully. Atropine should be applied topically into the eye two to three times daily to maintain pupillary dilatation and prevent the development of anterior synechiae.

Chapter 7

# *Intensive Care*

Intensive care is the term used to describe the nursing and treatment of a critically ill animal. The animals to whom this is applied are so ill that they would not survive without constant attention and regular interference to maintain their body function. It is applicable not only to acute trauma cases but also to surgical cases before and after major surgery and to medical cases.

Intensive care is designed to replace the normal homeostatic mechanisms of the body, which at the time, for whatever reason, are unable to function. Normally the body constantly monitors its own function and then automatically makes adjustments according to the information gained from this continuous surveillance. Regular monitoring and continual adjustment of the treatment regime thus form the basis of all intensive care. This continuous care must go on until the animal's condition is stable.

Good nursing is often the most important factor in deciding the outcome of the patient and ensures that the full significance of any changes in the animal's condition is understood. Experience is extremely valuable, and a visit to another establishment that has intensive care facilities is always worthwhile, particularly when first setting up a system in a practice.

The main requirement of intensive care is not elaborate facilities, but round-the-clock care of the patient. Although in the human field intensive care is synonymous with sophisticated and expensive equipment, a high standard of intensive care can still be applied to the sick animal with no more equipment than is found in the average veterinary practice. It is, however, extremely labour-intensive, since experienced nursing is required to care for the patient for 24 hours a day. Regular and frequent input from the veterinarian responsible for the case is also essential. This degree of care is difficult to maintain during the day in a busy practice; it is even more difficult to maintain at night, when those involved have to do a full day's work again the next day. However, the majority of veterinary patients do not require long periods of intensive care, and, although it often relies on good will, determination to see a patient survive usually keeps the team going. It does mean, however, that if there is normally no provision for night staff, there is a limit as to how many patients can be monitored intensively, particularly in the smaller practices.

The real cost of intensive care is considerable and may prove prohibitive; the decision to go ahead can only be made on the merits of each case. There is no doubt, however, that intensive care can be extremely rewarding.

The moral issues must not be forgotten, and the quality of life that the animal is likely to experience if it recovers should be taken into account. Euthanasia must still be considered an option in such cases.

## EQUIPMENT AND FACILITIES

### The room and general equipment

The actual room chosen will obviously depend on the premises involved. It is most important that the intensive care area is regularly frequented under normal circumstances and is not out of the way and easily forgotten, or the attending nurse will become bored and demoralized. It must also be comfortable and pleasant enough to stay in for long periods of time. A place near the coffee room or equivalent often provides the most satisfactory arrangement. All members of the practice will then inevitably take an interest in the progress of the animal, and the necessary care is far easier to provide. Equally, the chosen place must not mean that the normal running of the practice is totally disrupted. For this reason, the operating theatre or consulting room is quite unsuitable. Practices which have a post-anaesthetic recovery room can most effectively use a section of this for intensive care, but it is only the large institutions which can provide a special intensive care unit with staff always employed for the full 24 hours. The intensive care room should have good access to drugs and other equipment.

The intensive care patient should be nursed where it can easily be seen and reached from all sides. In general this means that a table is most suitable for those cases requiring constant attention. It is very difficult to monitor and treat an animal lying in the back of a kennel, particularly if it is at floor level. Ideally, as the patient improves and becomes more mobile it should be moved from its table to a kennel while still receiving constant attention. This is easily established in premises where the recovery room is used for intensive care, since there should already be kennels with easy access. Where no such arrangements exist, some sort of portable kennel will need to be set up in the designated intensive care area once the animal becomes more mobile. This allows for the transition from 24 hour care to the intermittent attention that the animal will receive once it is returned to the regular kennels.

Good lighting, heating and ventilation are essential. A telephone (with a list of the important numbers) or other means of contacting help in an emergency must be within easy reach. A clock with a second hand is also a vital piece of equipment. Some comfort for the attending nurse is of great benefit, especially during periods when only one person is present. A comfortable chair, reading material, means of making coffee/tea and a radio or cassette player go a long way towards making the night shift tolerable. Television is too distracting to be encouraged.

The debilitated animal is more susceptible to infection than the healthy one. The intensive care patient also has numerous routes of entry for bacteria, such as intravenous lines, and extreme care is necessary to prevent infection developing. Full-time medical intensive care wards operate under near-operating-theatre conditions to prevent establishment of nosocomial infections. While this is not feasible in the average practice, protective clothing contaminated from other animals should be removed before the intensive care patient is handled, and good personal cleanliness adhered to while nursing the patient.

A rota should always be drawn up to provide the nursing care. Veterinary supervision must be included in this rota at specific times, so that the lay staff know when the treatment will be reassessed. Although 24 hour nursing is not economical use of a veterinarian's time, so much can be learned during a spell of intensive care that it is worth including veterinarians on the duty rota for some periods.

**Specific veterinary equipment**

Nothing beyond the ordinary is required to apply the principles of intensive care but the essential items must be available at all times so that they are immediately to hand whenever the need arises. There is no time for preparation when a trauma case is admitted. Ideally the equipment should all be kept ready in the recovery or intensive care room.

*Stethoscope and thermometer*

Much of intensive care relies on good clinical examination, and the usual tools of the trade are required.

### Oxygen supply

Many patients in intensive care will require oxygen administration for a period of time. This can be supplied by mask, tracheostomy or endotracheal tube as appropriate. An oxygen cage is ideal but rarely available due to cost. Paediatric incubators often have a facility for providing oxygen-enriched air and are excellent for small patients. Oxygen is supplied either from cylinders or a pipeline system. The oxygen supply on an anaesthetic machine is often the most easily obtainable source, but a single oxygen cylinder with a two stage regulator or a regulator that incorporates a flow meter (*Fig.* 7.1) is quite sufficient as long as it can be connected to a means of providing IPPV.

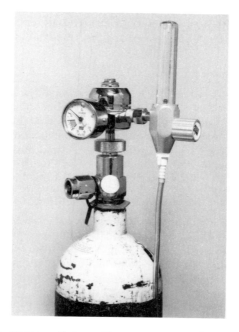

*Fig.* 7.1. An oxygen cylinder with a pressure regulator incorporating a flow-meter.

### Emergency resuscitation kit

Emergency cardiopulmonary resuscitation (*see* Chapter 8) is more likely to be required for the intensive care patient than for any other veterinary case. The kit should include a box containing a small range of endotracheal tubes with connectors, means of supplying IPPV with oxygen and drugs suitable for treating cardiac arrest. These are outlined in *Table* 8.3. An instruction sheet on dosage and course of action should be included (*see Table* 8.4). It is essential that all personnel likely to be called to deal with an emergency understand the system so that there is no confusion when time is critical.

### Sterile equipment for intravenous infusion

Placement of indwelling intravenous catheters is essential. Fluid and electrolyte replacement, and in some cases calories, must be provided by continuous intravenous infusion. These cannot be given through a needle since this will damage the vein, resulting in perivascular injection and local tissue damage. An indwelling catheter also provides ready access to the vein should this be required in an emergency, and removes the need for repeated venepuncture for drug administration. The technique of intravenous catheterization and details of the equipment required are described in Chapter 8.

### Sterile kit for urinary catheterization

The urinary bladder should be catheterized in all animals undergoing intensive care. Urine must be collected so that urine output can be measured. In addition, retention with overflow is prevented and the bladder can be emptied without the animal becoming soiled with urine. The necessary equipment and the techniques for placement of the various types of catheter are described in Chapter 8.

### Equipment for a chest drain and a tracheostomy tube

One of the major indications for veterinary intensive care is the animal that has a chest injury, or has had thoracic surgery, and requires repeated or continuous suction of air or fluid from the thoracic cavity in order to maintain adequate pulmonary ventilation. The equipment required and the technique of inserting a chest drain are described in Chapter 8.

### Means of applying suction

Suction may be required to aspirate the pleural cavity or to clear the airways. Mechanical electrically powered suction is by far the best apparatus for this purpose, and is well worth the initial outlay. Alternatively, a large syringe, tubing and a three-way stopcock (so that the syringe can be emptied without removing the tubing) can be used. However, it is much more laborious, and not suitable where continuous suction is required, as for instance in a pneumothorax with a continuous leak.

## *Drugs*

Drugs that are likely to be required in addition to those provided for emergency resuscitation include analgesics, fluids for intravenous use, sedatives and tranquillizers, antibiotics, diuretics and steroids. Their use is discussed below in the section on treatment.

## *Heating pads and insulation*

Blankets, plastic bubbles, space blankets and some form of thermostatically controlled heating pad will be required to maintain adequate body temperature.

## *Basic laboratory facilities*

Some laboratory back-up is required for monitoring the intensive care patient; at the very least this should include a microhaematocrit centrifuge so that PCV can be measured. A spectrophotometer for measurement of plasma proteins is also most valuable.

## *Other more sophisticated equipment*

More extensive laboratory facilities, an ECG, equipment for measuring arterial blood pressure and an automatic infusion pump are all useful additions to the basic requirements of intensive care. All of these are discussed in greater detail in the section on monitoring.

## GENERAL CARE OF THE ANIMAL

### General well-being

### *Position*

Physiologically, it is best to nurse the animal supported on its brisket, so that neither lung suffers from hypostatic congestion. However, it is very difficult to support an animal in this position for long periods, and the best alternative is to allow it to lie on its side and turn it at regular intervals. A record should be kept of when the animal is turned so that it is performed regularly. In most cases turning every 2–4 hours is adequate.

### *Cleanliness and comfort*

The animal must be kept clean by washing or grooming so that it is comfortable. Staining from urine or faeces will scald the skin and must be removed immediately. Even if the animal is not receiving anything by mouth, its sense of well-being will be improved if the mouth is rinsed out regularly with a little water. The nostrils and eyes should be kept clean and moist. Regardless of what is used to maintain body temperature, the animal should lie on a warm, comfortable and easily cleaned surface. Vetbed® is ideal since it fulfills all these criteria. It has the additional advantage that any fluid soaks down into the base so that the animal remains relatively dry.

### Temperature

The critically ill animal is unlikely to be able to maintain normal body temperature, and hypothermia is always a potential hazard. It is important to maintain a high ambient temperature in the intensive care room since this will help to prevent excessive heat loss. Blankets can be used if necessary but they make it difficult to see the animal and to maintain intravenous lines and catheters. Plastic bubbles (*Fig.* 7.2) have been found most effective in maintaining body temperature and do not impair visibility of the animal. Heating pads can, of course, help to maintain body temperature, but extreme care must be taken to ensure that these are not too hot, as the unconscious or comatosed animal is unable to move and may be badly burned. Insulation, particularly from a metal surface, is most important, and again Vetbed provides an ideal surface for the animal to lie on. The patient should

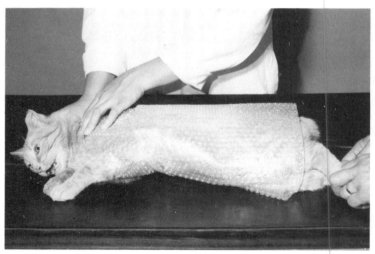

*Fig.* 7.2. Plastic bubbles provide a cheap and effective means of maintaining body temperature.

also be kept as dry as possible, since a wet animal will lose heat through the latent heat of vaporization.

## TLC

A little 'tender loving care' goes a long way. Time spent petting and talking to a sick animal is time well spent, and undoubtedly improves its sense of well-being. Hand feeding often helps the reluctant animal to start eating and may reduce the convalescent period substantially.

### Care of intravenous lines

During intensive care intravenous lines may be required for many days. It is absolutely essential that they are placed and maintained under aseptic conditions. The catheter itself should be covered with sterile gauze, held in place with bandages and extension tubing used for injections and handling (*Fig.* 7.3). This should help maintain asepsis of the venepuncture site. The dressing should be changed daily, the area cleaned with an organic iodine solution and the site inspected. If there are any signs of phlebitis the catheter should be changed, otherwise it is generally better to leave it in place so that accessible veins are not traumatized more than is necessary.

Intravenous catheters should be flushed regularly at least two to four times daily with heparinized saline (2 units per ml) to maintain their patency. Even when fluids flow through them continuously fibrin builds up on the catheter surface. Regular flushing will not prevent this deposition on the outside of the catheter but does help to maintain its patency.

Damaged catheters that have kinked or are leaking should be removed and replaced at once. It is possible for a damaged catheter to break off at the hub, disappear into the bloodstream and become lodged in a tissue where it may cause damage.

### Care of the respiratory system

#### Maintenance of the airway

A patent airway must be maintained at all times. The nose, mouth and pharynx must be kept clear of any secretions or vomit. The head and neck must be positioned in such a way that there is no constriction of the airway. Endotracheal tubes must be cleaned regularly. However, if tracheal intubation is required for any length of time, a tracheostomy should be employed. Tracheostomy is also required for any patient with acute upper airway obstruction. A tracheostomy tube requires careful attention since it entirely negates the animal's own protective

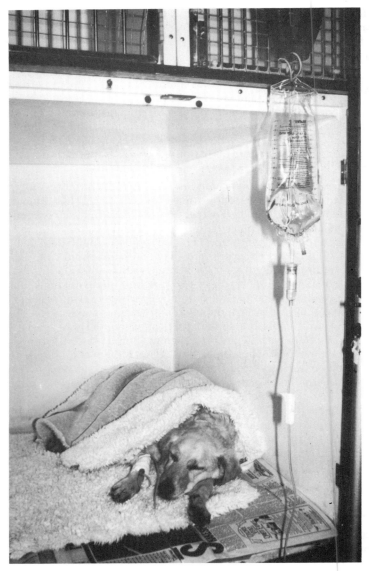

*Fig.* 7.3. Intravenous catheters should be bandaged and maintained as aseptically as possible.

reflexes. It should be flushed with a few millilitres of sterile saline at least two to four times daily, and sucked out immediately afterwards. If fibrin builds up excessively the tube must be changed before the airway becomes blocked.

### Care of the chest drain

A chest drain must be inserted and maintained under aseptic conditions. As with intravenous catheters the point of insertion should be kept covered, and connecting tubing used for access. The site should be checked and cleansed daily. Regular or continuous suction is usually sufficient to maintain patency of the tubing.

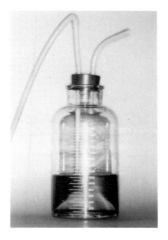

*Fig.* 7.4. An underwater seal. Suction can be applied to the short tube. The longer tube is connected to the chest drain. The water will rise a short way up the vertical arm due to the subatmospheric pressure in the chest.

The chest drain must *always* be connected to a one-way valve or be clamped off to prevent the development of a potentially fatal pneumothorax. The most effective one-way valve is the underwater seal (*Fig.* 7.4). This makes use of the fact that water will only rise a small distance up the tube in the bottle provided that the animal is at least 1·2 m above the bottle. If the bottle is raised higher than this, there is a danger that water will be sucked into the chest. The advantage of this system is that it supplies a great deal of information about conditions in the chest. This is discussed fully in the section on monitoring. With the underwater seal most animals can expel some air or fluid from the pleural cavity even when suction is not applied. The disadvantage of this system is that the animal must be kept still so that it does not become detached from the valve, or move to a level at which the water is sucked into the chest. This may necessitate tranquillization. Another one-way valve that can be used to seal the drain is the Heimlich valve (*Fig.* 7.5). This is an effective seal through which suction can be applied. It is small enough to be strapped to the side of larger dogs so that the animal can be mobile. However, most small animals are unable to expel pleural air or fluid through this without the aid of suction, and it simply acts as a seal through which suction can be applied intermittently without the need for sealing and unsealing the chest drain each time. It is too large to be useful in cats and small dogs. In these the tubing must be clamped between each chest aspiration.

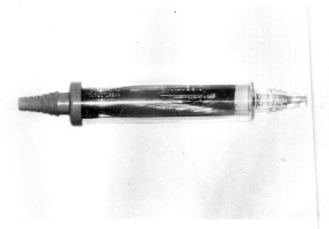

*Fig.* 7.5. A Heimlich valve can be attached to a chest drain to provide a one-way seal. The valve consists of an open ended cylinder of soft rubber within an outer protective case.

Mechanical suction should always be applied via a Heimlich valve or water trap as a safety measure to prevent excessive suction being applied to the chest. Where continuous suction is required it is most satisfactory to use the water trap. The animal already has to remain immobile for attachment of the suction apparatus, and information on the progress of the suction is continuously obvious from a glance at the water trap. Where a syringe is used it is easier to aspirate directly from the chest drain. Care must be taken not to allow air to enter the chest when the syringe is attached.

## Care of urinary catheters

Strict asepsis is required in the use of urinary catheters. Once inserted, it is preferable to leave catheters in place rather than traumatizing the urethra by frequent catheterization. Where at all possible, a self-retaining Foley catheter should be used, as it is very much easier to maintain in position that the conventional urinary catheter. Such catheters can be safely left for several days provided they remain patent. It may be helpful to flush them with a little sterile saline once or twice a day to prevent them from becoming blocked. Cats and male dogs present a problem, since it is not possible to obtain Foley catheters long enough for male dogs or small enough for cats. The Jackson cat catheter for male cats has a hub designed for suturing to the sheath, and ordinary catheters can generally also be sutured to the sheath or vulva (*see* Chapter 8).

The vulva or sheath should be cleansed daily to help maintain as near asepsis as possible around the urinary catheter.

## Management of pain

This is a particularly important aspect of intensive care of the traumatized and postoperative patient. Head injuries preclude the use of opiates, but all other trauma cases benefit from adequate analgesia. Assessment of the degree of pain, and administration of analgesics, is the dual responsibility of the veterinarian and the attending nurse. Considerable knowledge of what to expect is helpful, since such assessment is subjective and relies heavily on past experience.

## MONITORING

Monitoring is the essence of good intensive care. It provides an early warning system whereby changes in the animal's condition are spotted as soon as they occur, so that treatment can be adjusted accordingly. This should prevent the development of major problems, or at least ensure that they are treated as soon as they arise.

It is essential that a written record be kept, and that measurements be made at regular intervals. It is vital that trends, not just isolated facts, are recorded. A further advantage of written records is that information about the patient is easily passed on to the next nurse and to the attending veterinarian. Monitoring should be performed at specified time intervals of between 5 and 20 minutes, depending on the condition of the patient. It is much easier for nursing staff to carry out regular monitoring if a time interval is specified. Some sort of chart, with sections to fill in, also ensures that all the required measurements are carried out (*Table* 7.1).

*Table 7.1.* **Intensive care chart**

ANIMAL and date:
Prescriptions:

| time | pulse | respiration | temp. | urine | fluids | drugs | lab. | radiog. | comments |
|------|-------|-------------|-------|-------|--------|-------|------|---------|----------|
|      |       |             |       |       |        |       |      |         |          |
|      |       |             |       |       |        |       |      |         |          |
|      |       |             |       |       |        |       |      |         |          |
|      |       |             |       |       |        |       |      |         |          |
|      |       |             |       |       |        |       |      |         |          |
|      |       |             |       |       |        |       |      |         |          |

Parameters to monitor are set out below. Most of these require no more than good clinical observation and a little attention to detail, particularly in the record keeping. Each parameter must be recorded, but none should be assessed in isolation. Changes in the state of the animal since the previous observations were made should be noted. In this way the progress of the animal is continually assessed.

## Pulse

Pulse rate and quality should be recorded frequently and at regular intervals. This will provide a great deal of information about the cardiovascular system. For instance, the very fact that the peripheral pulses may be difficult to find is useful information and should be recorded. It suggests that peripheral circulation is poor and that circulatory support is required. Pulse rate is also informative. For instance, an increase in rate may indicate hypovolaemia, hypoxia, pain or sepsis.

## Respiration

Respiratory rate and character should be recorded at the same time intervals as the pulse. It is worthwhile standing back and making a subjective assessment of the respiratory pattern as well as recording more objective information. Does the animal appear to have difficulty breathing? Does the chest wall get sucked in when the animal inspires, suggesting that there is partial upper airway obstruction?

Respiratory rate is a particularly helpful parameter to record. An increase in rate may indicate pain, hypoxia, sepsis or deteriorating pulmonary function. Conversely, a decrease in rate towards normal, coupled with an improved tidal volume, is usually a good prognostic sign.

Auscultation should be performed regularly to provide information about the lung field. Daily or twice-daily radiographic examination of the chest is indicated if there are any signs of chest pathology.

Where pneumo- or hydrothorax is being treated with a chest drain and suction, information about the thoracic cavity can be gleaned from the behaviour of an underwater seal. The water column reflects the intrapleural pressure. In normal circumstances the top of the column is a few centimetres above the surface of the water and swings a further few centimetres up and down with breathing. Should the column swing more than this it indicates that air is present in the pleural cavity and needs to be removed. Both air and fluid may be discharged from the drain at expiration. The underwater seal is particularly useful where air is concerned as bubbles will be seen. Suction should be applied to the chest drain at regular intervals and a record made of what is aspirated. The frequency of suction depends entirely on the need, and continuous suction may be required in some instances. Where this is the case, the volume of fluid extracted in unit time is recorded. the number of bubbles produced per minute is also recorded where appropriate.

### Temperature

A clinical thermometer can be used per rectum to monitor temperature at regular intervals. A thermocouple probe (*Fig.* 7.6) is to be preferred, however, as it provides a continuous read-out without the need to keep reinserting the probe. It is also possible to measure near core temperatures by inserting a longer probe deeper into the body, for instance into the oesophagus. This provides a more accurate assessment of true body temperature and metabolic rate than peripheral temperature, which is too dependent on local blood flow. Measurement of core and peripheral temperature provides a useful guide to peripheral blood flow. Normally rectal and oesophageal temperature are only 1–2° C apart. Where peripheral blood flow is reduced, as in a shocked animal, this difference may be greater. A graphic record of temperature is particularly useful so that trends can be seen. This is essential when alterations to body temperature are

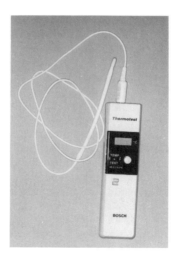

*Fig.* 7.6. A thermocouple probe provides a continuous read out of the animal's temperature. The probe may be inserted further than a thermometer, permitting measurement of near core temperature.

being made by adjusting insulation and heating pads and by giving warmed fluids, as the results are slow to materialize.

A further, if somewhat subjective, assessment of peripheral temperature and thus peripheral circulation is simply to feel the paws and ears. If these are strikingly cold to the touch it is essential that both circulation and actual temperature are improved.

## Mucous membranes

The colour should be recorded. This is a subjective assessment and cannot be relied upon to a great extent; however, it is useful in extreme circumstances and when assessing response to treatment. Hypoxia does not always produce cyanosis, but where cyanosis is present prompt treatment is indicated. In these circumstances the mucous membrane colour provides a useful monitor.

The mucous membranes should also be palpated. Dry, cold membranes usually indicate a shocked patient in need of circulatory support with intravenous fluids.

Capillary refill time is worth noting, although it can be misleading, and must be assessed with other clinical signs. It is measured by applying digital pressure to the mucous membranes of the gum or tongue until the area blanches, and noting the time taken for the capillaries to refill when the pressure is released. Normal reaction is almost instantaneous. A slow refill indicates poor capillary perfusion and that fluid therapy is required. A fast refill does not always mean that all is well, however; it may be seen when cardiac output is poor and there is peripheral pooling of blood.

## Urinary output

Measurement of the volume of urine passed in unit time is one of the most simple but useful techniques used in monitoring the intensive care patient. Assuming that there is no primary renal disease, urine production indicates adequate perfusion of the kidneys. If this is the case, it follows that the rest of the body is also adequately perfused. Oliguria or anuria is a serious affair which must be investigated and treated as soon as possible. The former is particularly difficult to spot unless output is closely monitored.

Urine is collected into a bag from the urinary catheter and the volume measured at regular intervals. Hourly assessment is advisable where there is any doubt that urine output is insufficient. This is performed either by weighing the bag and noting the difference from the previous time, or by emptying the bag into a measuring cylinder each time the volume is recorded. Urine production of less than

$0.5–1.0$ ml kg$^{-1}$ h$^{-1}$ indicates that output is too low and that specific treatment is indicated.

## Fluid output

Abnormal losses of any other fluid such as vomit, diarrhoea, pleural, peritoneal or respiratory secretions should be recorded.

## Fluid input

In the same way that the volume of fluid voided from the body is measured, so the input must also be monitored. This simply entails keeping a careful record of how much has been given in the previous hour. This is most easily performed by weighing the infusion bag with a spring balance, as it is impossible to estimate accurately how much of a collapsible bag of fluid has been used in any other way. With faster infusions, the drip rate is counted regularly (*Table* 7.2), unless an infusion pump is available in which case the setting must be confirmed periodically. It is most important to know the volume of fluid administered so that response to treatment can be assessed and the infusion rate altered as necessary. The type of fluid administered must also be recorded. If intravenous feeding is in progress, the rate of calorie input should also be noted.

*Table 7.2.* **Guide to infusion rates**

---

Most standard size infusion sets in England produce 20 drops to one ml

'Mini' drip sets produce 60 drops per ml

Standard sets:
   $10\,\text{ml}\,\text{kg}^{-1}\,\text{h}^{-1} = 3$ drops kg$^{-1}$ min$^{-1}$ ... for 25 kg dog = 80 drops/min
                                                       for 4 kg dog (cat) = 13 drops/min
   $30\,\text{ml}\,\text{kg}^{-1}\,\text{h}^{-1} = 10$ drops kg$^{-1}$ min$^{-1}$ ... for 25 kg dog = 250 drops/min
                                                       for 4 kg dog (cat) = 40 drops/min
   $90\,\text{ml}\,\text{kg}^{-1}\,\text{h}^{-1} = 30$ drops kg$^{-1}$ min$^{-1}$ ... for 25 kg dog = 750 drops/min
                                                       for 4 kg dog (cat) = 120 drops/min

'Mini' sets
   $10\,\text{ml}\,\text{kg}^{-1}\,\text{h}^{-1} = 10$ drops kg$^{-1}$ min$^{-1}$ ... for 4 kg dog (cat) = 40 drops/min
   $30\,\text{ml}\,\text{kg}^{-1}\,\text{h}^{-1} = 30$ drops kg$^{-1}$ min$^{-1}$ ... for 4 kg dog (cat) = 120 drops/min
   $90\,\text{ml}\,\text{kg}^{-1}\,\text{h}^{-1} = 90$ drops kg$^{-1}$ min$^{-1}$ ... for 4 kg dog (cat) = 360 drops/min

---

The current rate of infusion must be closely monitored so that it keeps as close as possible to that prescribed. Sudden fast infusions due to changes in the animal's position must be avoided. Cessation of infusion due to blocked lines must be spotted and rectified immediately. Automatic infusion pumps are most useful in these circumstances, but are inevitably expensive. Paediatric infusion sets provide a safety factor in tiny patients. The cuvette is filled from the main infusion bag so that, should there be a sudden surge, only that in the cuvette will be infused, not the contents of the whole bag. It is important to close the junction between bag and cuvette, however, or a false sense of security will prevail!

**Central venous pressure**

The technique for measuring central venous pressure (CVP) is described in Chapter 8. It simply involves the measurement of venous pressure close to the right atrium. It provides useful information regarding the animal's fluid needs, since it is related to the filling of the vascular bed. It also provides information about the ability of the heart to handle intravenous infusion. Appreciation of absolute CVP value is less important than examination of any change. A low CVP, below zero or less than about $5 \, cmH_2O$, indicates that the animal is hypovolaemic, and that the heart is not overloaded. A sudden rise in CVP indicates adequate infusion or that the heart (the right side at least) is unable to cope with the infusion. In this case the infusion should be slowed. It is a useful additional guide to the progress of intravenous infusion. The response of CVP to a small rapid infusion (say 15–30 ml/kg over 1–3 minutes) is often most illuminating: if CVP rises momentarily but falls back to where it started the animal requires more fluid and there is little danger of overloading the heart. However, if the CVP rises substantially and remains high for several minutes after such an infusion, it indicates that the vascular system is adequately filled and that infusion may be slowed. If there is a rapid and sustained rise after the test infusion it indicates that the heart is unable to cope with the load and infusion must be stopped. It may suggest that some cardiac support is required.

**General demeanour of the animal**

The animal's mental state is a useful guide to some aspects of the physiological state of the body. Restlessness and tachypnoea may be caused by pain, hypoxia, developing sepsis and chest pathology. Loss of consciousness or mental stupor may indicate shock or hypoxia. General weakness may be a sign of hypokalaemia. All these factors, with particular attention being paid to any changes that are seen, should be recorded. Signs of pain and the response to analgesics should also be noted, so that pain relief can be provided at appropriate intervals.

## Packed cell volume and plasma proteins

These should be monitored at regular intervals as they provide another guide to the animal's fluid balance. The normal range of PP in the dog is 55–85 g/l. Older animals (with an increased globulin fraction from repeated antigenic stimulation) will tend to have values at the upper end of the range. The normal range in the cat is 55–85 g/l. The animal that is short of both water and water with electrolytes will have an elevated PP concentration due to the loss of non-protein extracellular fluid. After haemorrhage the concentration will be reduced.

Normal PCV in the dog is 40 l/l and in the cat 37 l/l. PCV is less reliable than PP as a guide to the degree of hydration, since recent haemorrhage and anaemia may alter the haematocrit without there being any change in fluid and electrolyte balance. Regular assessment of these parameters viewed together is particularly helpful when the response to long term fluid infusion is assessed. If the PCV and PP fall too low, fluid infusion should be slowed or replaced with a colloid infusion that will maintain colloid oncotic pressure, and retain fluid in the circulation. If PCV and PP remain high, it suggests that fluid infusion could be more aggressive.

The techniques employed in measurement of PCV and PP concentration are described in Chapter 8.

## Electrocardiography

This is the first of the more sophisticated investigations involving equipment which is not absolutely essential, but is extremely useful if available. A simple pulse rate monitor that bleeps at each QRS complex but does not show the PQRS trace is not worth having in intensive care. The rate may continue unaltered and lull the clinician into a false sense of security while serious changes in the PQRS complex go undetected. Dysrhythmias and changes in the PQRS pattern are not uncommon in the intensive care patient. Hypoxia and electrolyte imbalance will produce changes, particularly in the T wave. Unless the leads have been very carefully placed it is usually more important to note changes rather than the absolute pattern of the PQRS complex. A diagnosis may not be reached, but a warning that all is not well is sounded so that other investigations can be made. Administration of oxygen may be all that is required.

## Arterial blood pressure

Arterial blood pressure measurement is again not essential but provides additional useful information.

Coupled with measurement of urinary output and CVP, arterial blood pressure completes the picture for thorough cardiovascular monitoring. Low blood pressure is not unusual in the intensive care patient, and since many systems in the body, notably the kidneys, depend on adequate blood pressure for normal function, it is pertinent to try to maintain a mean arterial blood pressure above 60 mmHg. Fluid infusion, and possibly catecholamine therapy, may be required to achieve this. However, it is difficult to detect the need for catecholamines without the facility of arterial blood pressure measurement. It is also a particularly valuable parameter to measure when assessing their effects. While few practices can afford the luxury of an electronic system using strain gauge transducers, a simple aneroid manometer which gives mean pressure only (*Fig.* 7.7) connected to an arterial line is cheap and most effective. Cannulation of an artery is described in Chapter 8.

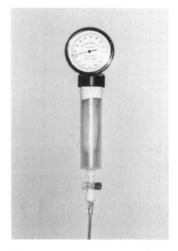

*Fig.* 7.7. The Pressurveil system provides a convenient means of connecting a simple aneroid manometer to an arterial cannula to measure blood pressure.

Indirect monitors using a cuff and a pulse detector (*Fig.* 7.8) are also available. These have the advantage of being non-invasive, but they do not give a continuous record. The cuff must be of an appropriate size for the animal concerned and is inflated and slowly released each time a reading is made.

## Arterial blood gas analysis and electrolyte concentration

These measurements can only be made with the aid of sophisticated and expensive equipment. Results from such analyses are most

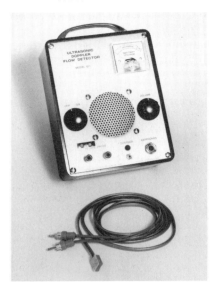

*Fig.* 7.8. A Doppler blood pressure monitor provides a non-invasive method for measuring arterial blood pressure.

instructive, but unless known within a few minutes of sampling are not too useful because the situation is likely to change rapidly. If, however, there is access to such information it is particularly helpful for guidance in the type of fluid to administer. Many animals in intensive care are acidotic, but it is difficult to diagnose this without measurement of blood pH. Without such information treatment is empirical. Similarly, electrolyte imbalances are notoriously difficult to detect on clinical grounds alone.

## TREATMENT

It is beyond the scope of this book to detail treatment for every kind of intensive care case. Indeed, treatment of these patients must be made to meet individual requirements. A few general principles are outlined below.

### Fluid therapy

The major requirement of the intensive care patient is for adequate fluid therapy. Fortunately, in all but the cases with renal disease, as long as the volume is adequate, it is remarkable how the kidney will compensate for errors in composition. This is particularly important where it is not possible to measure plasma electrolytes and pH. When there is kidney failure, however, extreme care must be taken not to overtransfuse.

Fluid requirements can be divided into two major groups: replacement and maintenance.

### Replacement

The basic principle behind replacement therapy is that the fluid lost should be replaced with as near as possible the same type of fluid. It is therefore necessary to assess both the quality and the quantity of what has been lost.

Replacement therapy for the intensive care patient will generally be required to treat actual or impending hypovolaemic shock. This is discussed in detail in Chapter 2. Such therapy must be given by the intravenous route for it to be effective. Many of the symptoms of shock are the same, regardless of the underlying cause, but it is necessary to establish the cause in order to provide the most rational treatment. History is the most useful guide for the initial treatment. If the animal has recently suffered trauma the most likely cause is haemorrhage, while mixed fluid and electrolyte depletion will be the result of systemic disease such as gastroenteritis. PCV and PP estimation may prove to be the most informative specific investigations. PCV and PP will be normal or low after haemorrhage and high after water and electrolyte depletion.

### Quality

Haemorrhage should, in theory, be replaced with whole blood. In practice this is often difficult, due to problems of collection, storage and cross-matching. Alternatives to blood are plasma (which is often less practical to provide than whole blood), colloidal solutions such as Haemaccel (Hoechst) or dextrans, and electrolyte solutions. The disadvantage of using electrolyte solutions is that they do not stay within the vascular bed, but diffuse into the rest of the ECF space so that approximately three times the volume of blood lost is required to re-expand the circulation. If substantial blood loss (more than 25 per cent of the circulating blood volume) is replaced in this way, colloid oncotic pressure will fall and the extravascular spaces will be overloaded, resulting in oedema. The haemoglobin concentration will also be markedly reduced, resulting in decreased oxygen carrying capacity of the blood. Colloidal solutions, including plasma, do not diffuse out of the circulation into the rest of the ECF, and are therefore a better alternative after substantial blood loss. However, these too do not have oxygen carrying capacity, and losses of more than 50 per cent of the circulating volume need to be replaced at least in part with whole blood. There is considerable evidence to suggest that it is better to use part blood and part non-blood products (such as electrolytes and colloids) for treatment of haemorrhage.

Mixed water and electrolyte depletion require replacement with electrolyte solutions. The exact nature of the electrolyte solution can be deduced from the history and knowledge of the underlying disease process. Laboratory tests, where these can be obtained, are particularly helpful to indicate the more subtle electrolyte imbalances. In general, losses due to vomiting, diarrhoea, peritoneal and pleural effusions, toxaemia and septicaemia will be isotonic and are best replaced with a balanced electrolyte solution such as lactated Ringer's. Where losses are severe and cardiovascular collapse imminent, plasma replacement fluids should be used initially, so that the circulation is restored as quickly as possible without fluid being lost into the tissues. The rest of the ECF can be restored more slowly once the circulation is in better condition.

Acidosis and hypokalaemia are the two most likely conditions that may need specific treatment over and above replacement fluids. These cannot be diagnosed with certainty without laboratory back-up but the history and clinical findings may be suggestive. Hyperventilation, when no other cause is detectable, suggests that the animal is acidotic, while generalized weakness and failure to respond as expected suggests that the animal is hypokalaemic. Up to 20–30 mmol/l KCl or 0·5–1·0 mmol/l $NaHCO_3$ can be added to the infusion as appropriate. Potassium should not be added to solutions given to animals with renal failure as they are likely to be hyperkalaemic.

Primary water depletion is unlikely to be a cause of hypovolaemic shock. Such depletion is borne by the whole body, not just the ECF, and signs due to dehydration of the CNS are usually seen first. Provision of daily requirements, as discussed below, must prevent such water depletion from developing.

*Quantity*

The history and severity of clinical signs are the best guides as to how much fluid should be given. Estimation of percentage dehydration is a useful, if subjective, additional guide and is used to calculate the initial volume to infuse as follows:

Bodyweight (kg) × % dehydration = litres of fluid required

Guidelines for the degree of dehydration assessed from the clinical examination are 5–6 per cent for mild dehydration, 8 per cent when it is moderate, 10 per cent when it is severe and 12–15 per cent when life-threatening. The most useful guide to the volume required, however, is the response to treatment.

If the depletion is considerable, the initial infusion should be given rapidly. Up to 90 ml/kg can be infused in the first hour. This must be closely monitored, ideally by measuring the CVP, to ensure that the circulation does not become overloaded. This rate of infusion is potentially dangerous and must be slowed as soon as possible, once improvement in the circulation is seen.

### Maintenance

The intensive care patient that is not taking any food or fluids by mouth must have the whole of its daily requirements provided parenterally. Maintenance fluids can be given by slow and continuous infusion, and the intravenous route is by far the most satisfactory for the purpose.

### Quality

The major component of the animal's daily requirement is water. Some sodium is also needed to replace normal losses. So-called fifth normal sodium chloride (0·18 per cent NaCl with 4 per cent dextrose) is ideal for the purpose. With regard to electrolytes, this solution is hypotonic, and thus provides mainly water. It is made up to the same osmolarity as plasma by the addition of dextrose so that it does not cause haemolysis when infused. The dextrose is metabolized and makes little long term contribution to plasma osmolarity.

Where there are continuing abnormal losses, as, for instance, in pleural effusion, these must also be made up. Such abnormal losses should normally be treated by using isotonic 'replacement' fluids.

Intensive care patients also require calories. The dextrose provided by maintenance fluids does not provide sufficient to prevent a negative energy balance from developing. One or two days without calorie supplement can be tolerated, but beyond this parenteral feeding is necessary. Commercially available high energy infusions can be given by intravenous infusion, and those containing glucose, fructose and essential amino acids (Vamin, Kabivitrum) or a fat emulsion (Intralipid, Kabivitrum) have been found adequate. The actual number of calories given is usually limited by the volume in which the infusion is administered, and there is no danger of giving too many calories unless the animal is overtransfused. Animals should be encouraged to eat as soon as possible, and fed little and often with tempting and highly digestible food.

*Quantity*

A normal dog or cat loses in the order of 40 ml/kg per day of water. Approximately half of this is lost in the urine, and the rest as so-called 'insensible losses' from the respiratory tract and in faeces. These losses continue when the animal is not eating or drinking, and must be provided parenterally. The fluid requirements of the intensive care patient are likely to be slightly higher than 40 ml/kg per day. Up to 80 ml/kg may be required for very small or young patients. Enough to maintain a urine output of at least 20 ml/kg per day should be given. In addition to the replacement of normal daily water requirements, the abnormal losses should be replaced with a volume of fluid that is equal to that lost.

**Oxygen**

Administration of oxygen is particularly valuable in patients with reduced lung volume or with poor peripheral perfusion. Although it is often regarded as emergency treatment, long term oxygen administration, by improving tissue oxygenation, may speed the animal's recovery and improve its well-being in a subtle manner. The practicalities of oxygen administration are described in Chaps 1 and 8.

**Analgesics and sedatives**

*Analgesics*

Many of the animals requiring intensive care will be in pain. This is obvious in the case of trauma or surgery, less so in the case of some systemic disease. Analgesia is an extremely important aspect of intensive care, both on humane grounds and also because, by improving the animal's sense of well-being, morbidity is reduced. The only absolute contraindication to the use of analgesics (particularly the opiates) is in head injury. Opiates raise intracranial pressure, and any analgesic may mask the development of neurological signs important for assessing and thus treating the underlying pathology.

Morphine is undoubtedly the most effective analgesic. Buprenorphine and pentazocine have the advantage of not falling under the jurisdiction of the Controlled Drugs regulations and are also extremely effective analgesics. It has been the authors' experience, however, that morphine is still superior for chest injury. Pethidine is considerably less effective in the dog and is very short acting. Methadone is effective for a relatively short period and offers no advantage over buprenorphine and pentazocine. All these can be given by intravenous or intramuscular injection.

Opiates are respiratory depressants, but cats and particularly dogs are not as susceptible to these effects as man. In cases of chest injury opiate analgesia will improve ventilation by reducing the pain.

Non-steroidal anti-inflammatory drugs are not such effective analgesics as the opiates. They are, therefore, less useful for intensive care.

Analgesics must be given as necessary by the attending nurse. A maximum dose (*see Table* 1.1) and a maximum frequency should be prescribed. In most circumstances opiates should not be given more than four-hourly.

### *Sedatives*

Some intensive care patients will require sedation so that intravenous lines, and more particularly chest drains, can be kept in place. It is better to avoid drugs such as acepromazine which have a hypotensive effect if the animal is at all hypovolaemic. Diazepam can be given intravenously to effect with little danger of cardiovascular depression. Doses of up to $1\,mg\ kg^{-1}\ h^{-1}$ can be used, although in general considerably less than this will be found adequate. Diazepam has a synergistic effect with opiates, and when the two are used in combination sedation and analgesia are particularly effective.

### Antibiotics

Broad spectrum antibiotics should always be given to all trauma and postoperative intensive care cases, and preferably to any others with indwelling catheters. These animals are particularly susceptible to infection. Ampicillin is generally the first choice. High doses are well tolerated, water-based solutions can be given by most routes, and it leaves the more exotic antibiotics for later use if necessary.

### Steroids

Cerebral oedema, from whatever cause, may benefit from steroid therapy. Dexamethasone 2–4 mg/kg four- to six-hourly for up to 3 days (the dose should then be reduced) may be beneficial.

The use of steroids in the shocked patient is discussed in Chapter 2.

### Diuretics

Diuretics have two main roles in the intensive care patient. The first is to encourage kidney function if renal failure is suspected. This is particularly relevant to acute pre-renal failure which has developed as a result of hypovolaemia, hypotension and inadequate perfusion. The second role is in the treatment of oedema, particularly cerebral and to a lesser extent pulmonary oedema.

Frusemide is the first line of treatment when attempting to establish urine output: 1–2 mg/kg intravenously are usually sufficient. If urine output is established it is essential that fluid therapy then keeps up with the urine output, or hypovolaemia will develop. Up to 5 mg/kg frusemide may be required to treat pulmonary and cerebral oedema.

Mannitol is the treatment of choice for reduction of cerebral oedema. Up to 1 g/kg as a 10 per cent solution is infused over 30 minutes, and can be repeated every 6–12 hours for 2–3 days if necessary. Care must be taken than the animal does not become dehydrated, and mannitol should not be used where cerebral haemorrhage is suspected.

## Vasoactive drugs

The use of both catecholamines and vasodilators is discussed in relation to the treatment of shock in Chapter 2.

In the intensive care patient a situation may arise where, in spite of the administration of an adequate volume of fluids, cardiac output is poor and hypotension persists. Infusion of an inotropic drug, given to effect, can be most beneficial.

Adrenaline may be used, but dopamine or dobutamine are probably more satisfactory as they improve myocardial contractility without either substantially increasing the heart rate or producing severe peripheral vasoconstriction. Doses are given in *Table* 7.3.

Table 7.3. **Drugs for cardiac support**

| | |
|---|---|
| Dobutamine | 10 μg/kg<br>(250 mg in 1 litre 5% dextrose<br>0·04 ml (1 drop) kg$^{-1}$ min$^{-1}$) |
| Dopamine | As for dobutamine |
| Adrenaline | 1:50 000 – give to effect<br>(dilute 1 ml 1:1000 to 50 ml with saline) |

# Chapter 8

# *Techniques*

Many of the techniques described in this chapter require an operator and at least one assistant. Care of the seriously injured animal calls for all the skills and cooperation that the veterinarian and nurse team can provide. Complete care of the critically ill animal cannot be performed by one person alone, and only immediate life-saving measures (such as intubation of the trachea) should be attempted single-handed.

## Endotracheal intubation

Intubation of the trachea is the first action required in the treatment of many seriously injured animals. It is essential that this is performed swiftly and without causing further injury to the patient. A reliable technique must be practised and used regularly, so that nothing unfamiliar is needed when emergency intubation is required.

Dogs and cats are not difficult to intubate unless injury to the face and jaw has changed the shape of the airways. Both species are most easily intubated with the help of an assistant.

A cuffed Magill tube (either plastic or red rubber) is most commonly available, and is quite satisfactory for dogs over 3–4 kg body weight. New Magill tubes are generally too long and should if necessary be cut to length so that dead space is kept to a minimum. Shortening the tube also prevents any chance of it entering a main bronchus which results in one side of the chest being unventilated. Ideally the tube should reach from the incisors to the point of the shoulder when measured against the animal before intubation. The tube should be lubricated and fitted with a connector before it is inserted. Cats and tiny dogs are best intubated with a plain tube. On cuffed tubes of 5 mm internal

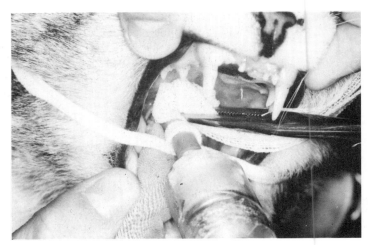

*Fig.* 8.1. The pharynx should be packed with gauze bandage to prevent aspiration of oral secretions when a non-cuffed tube is used.

diameter or less the cuff itself takes up a large proportion of the overall diameter so that an unnecessarily small airway is provided. If aspiration of mouth secretions is likely, the pharynx can be packed to provide a secure airway (*Fig.* 8.1). A slight leak around the tube is actually helpful when IPPV is required in really small animals since it prevents inadvertent overinflation of the lungs.

The animal, which is either anaesthetized or unconscious as a result of its injuries, is supported in lateral or sternal recumbency. The assistant grasps the back of the head with one hand and raises the head into a normal vertical position. The other hand is used to hold the upper jaw so that the operator inserting the tube can pull the lower jaw down and take hold of the tongue (*Fig.* 8.2). The tongue is then pulled out between the canine teeth and the tip pulled downwards. This action pulls the epiglottis forwards so that the entrance to the larynx can be exposed by gently pushing up the soft palate with the tip of the endotracheal tube. The tube is then pushed through the larynx and on into the trachea. No force is required; if difficulty is experienced once the tip of the tube is in the larynx it suggests that the tube is too large or that the tube is being pushed in the wrong direction. Once in place, the tube should be secured by tying a tape around its junction with the connector. This is then secured around the upper jaw, or around the back of the head in cats and short-nosed dogs.

This technique has the advantage that the operator controls the tongue and lower jaw, and has been found effective even in extreme

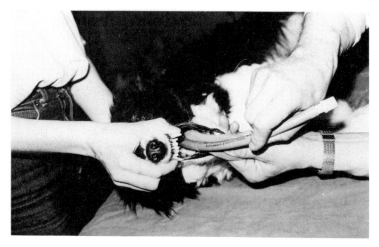

*Fig.* 8.2. Endotracheal intubation. The tongue is pulled down to hold the lower jaw. This also pulls the epiglottis forwards to expose the entrance to the larynx.

circumstances. If difficulty is experienced in exposing the larynx a laryngoscope should be used. The laryngoscope depresses the tongue and should on no account be used to immobilize the larynx itself as severe damage may result. If the condition of the animal permits it is particularly helpful to turn it on to its back and to lift the tongue. In this case the weight of the animal's head helps to expose the glottis (*Fig.* 8.3).

The same principles apply to the cat as to the dog, but the cat's larynx and trachea should be treated with even more respect. The cat has a powerful laryngeal reflex, and spasm is easily provoked by rough handling. It is also small and fragile so that minor damage may result in oedema and cause serious airway obstruction. The most common means of facilitating intubation in the anaesthetized cat is to depress the protective laryngeal reflex by spraying 1–2 per cent lignocaine on to the vocal cords before the tube is passed. This in itself provokes a reaction, and it is most important that whenever this technique is used sufficient time (30 s) is allowed for the local anaesthetic to take effect before any attempt is made to pass the tube. It is then necessary to wait until the cords open before the tube is pushed into the trachea. Exerting pressure on a closed glottis simply provokes spasm. If spasm were to occur, 2–3 mg (total dose in the cat) of suxamethonium should be given intravenously without delay, and the cat intubated and ventilated until spontaneous respiration returns. A 14 gauge needle can be used as a temporary tracheostomy if no other means of

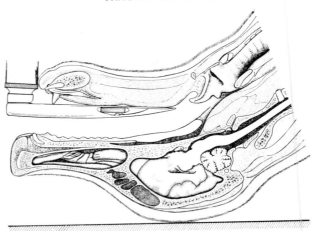

*Fig.* 8.3. The laryngoscope is used to depress the tongue. It should not be advanced further than depicted.

treatment is available. Laryngeal spasm is rarely a problem in the dog as tightly closed cords are not a common hazard of intubation.

Where only one person is available for intubation it is most satisfactory to use a mouth gag or, if necessary, a block of wood or a bandage to hold the mouth open. The tongue can then be manipulated in the same way as described above. This is most easily performed with the animal in lateral recumbency. Single-handed intubation using a laryngoscope is best performed with the animal on its back. Intubation may be extremely difficult in the severely dyspnoeic animal and assistance, from the unskilled if necessary, is highly desirable.

Animals who are to undergo surgery to correct severe jaw injuries may be intubated via a pharyngostomy incision. This will improve access to the mouth and will allow alignment of the jaws to be checked so that a correct bite is restored. The endotracheal tube can then be replaced with a pharyngostomy tube to provide an easy method of feeding.

After induction of anaesthesia and intubation a gag is inserted between the canine teeth. A gloved finger is then pushed into the piriform fossa to tent out the pharyngeal wall. A 1–2 cm skin incision is made in the overlying skin and a curved pair of artery forceps are introduced via this incision and pushed through the pharyngeal wall. The connector is temporarily removed and the cranial end of the endotracheal tube is grasped by the forceps and withdrawn through the pharyngostomy incision.

If required, after surgery, the endotracheal tube may be replaced by a plastic pharyngostomy tube or Foley catheter, pushed down the oesophagus. The caudal end of the tube should extend just beyond the cardia while the cranial end should be sutured to the skin. The position of the tube within the stomach should be checked radiographically, since an overlong tube will induce vomiting and an unduly short tube may result in regurgitation. Up to 100 ml of liquidized food should be fed 4–8 times a day, depending upon the size of the animal. The end of the tube is kept plugged between meals to prevent regurgitation, and the pharyngostomy wound is cleaned twice daily.

## Intravenous cannulation

Ready access to a vein for intravenous injection, infusion and blood withdrawal is essential in the treatment of the severely traumatized animal. An indwelling intravenous cannula should be placed as soon as possible after treatment begins. If placed under aseptic conditions, and maintained with care, such a cannula can be left *in situ* for many days so that further damage to veins is avoided and there is never any delay or difficulty in intravenous administration of drugs and fluids.

It is essential to use a cannula rather than a needle since a needle will damage the vein and result in perivascular injection. A cannula conforms more readily to the vein and stays in the lumen without unduly damaging its intima. Commercially available plastic cannulae come in many sizes and are ideal for use in animals.

Cannulae are supplied as either 'over the needle' or 'through the needle' versions (*Fig.* 8.4). The 'over the needle' variety is probably the easiest to use as it is inserted in a similar manner to a needle. Silicone catheters provoke the least tissue reaction, and if maintained

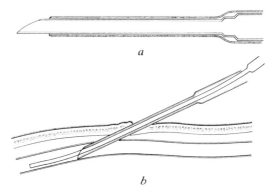

*Fig.* 8.4. *a*, 'Over the needle' cannula; *b*, 'through the needle' cannula.

under aseptic conditions, may be left *in situ* for many weeks. The more common Teflon or polyethylene catheters are, however, quite adequate for most veterinary purposes. Catheters with parallel walls rather than the tapered variety are the most satisfactory for small animal work. They have a tendency to kink where the hub joins the shaft of the catheter and need to be secured in place in such a way as to minimize this problem.

A list of recommended sizes is given in *Table* 8.1.

Table 8.1. **Intravenous cannulae**

| | | |
|---|---|---|
| Cephalic | | |
| Cats/small dogs | 22 G | 2·5 cm |
| Med. dogs | 20 G | 4 cm |
| Large dogs | 18 G | 5–8 cm |
| Jugular | | |
| Cats/small dogs | 20–18 G | 8–15 cm |
| Med. dogs | 16 G | 25 cm |
| Large dogs | 14 G | 30 cm |

A three-way stopcock is the most useful means of sealing the end of the catheter while still allowing easy access for infusions, injections or withdrawal of blood (*Fig.* 8.5*b*). This is particularly important in order to allow regular flushing of the cannula with heparinized saline (2 units per ml) to maintain its patency. A three-way stopcock may, however, be too bulky for the smaller patients, particularly if the cephalic vein is used. In this case a screw-on rubber bung (*Fig.* 8.5*a*) is the most satisfactory alternative. A needle can be inserted through the rubber for injections and blood withdrawal.

All the necessary equipment (*Table* 8.2) should be collected together before the animal is positioned for catheterization and the procedure started. The site is clipped and scrubbed as for surgery. Asepsis is most easily accomplished if sterile gloves are used, but a 'no touch' technique (where nothing that is to come into contact with the prepared site is touched) is adequate for short term cephalic cannulae. A small intradermal injection of local anaesthetic solution may be made over the intended site, but since this often appears more painful than insertion of the cannula itself, it is not essential. A 1–2 mm incision is then made in the skin with a no. 11 scalpel blade at the intended point of entry for the cannula. This facilitates the passage of the cannula through the skin, prevents kinking and ensures smooth intravenous puncture.

Cannulation of the cephalic vein with an 'over the needle' cannula is performed in a similar manner to intravenous injection with a needle, and the animal is positioned accordingly. The tip of the catheter is

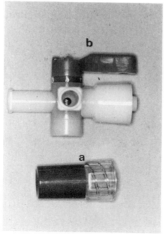

*Fig.* 8.5. a, A screw-on rubber bung used for sealing the end of an intravenous cannula in small dogs and cats. b, A three-way stopcock may be used in larger dogs.

*Table 8.2.* **Equipment for intravenous cannulation**

Skin prep. (e.g. organic iodine)
Surgical spirit
Local anaesthetic solution (2% lignocaine)
Scalpel blade, scissors
Heparin saline (2 units per ml)
Cannulae
Three-way stopcock or plug
Suture material and/or tape
Swabs and bandages
Sterile gloves
Sterile packs for 'cut down' should also contain drapes,
    artery forceps, tissue forceps and scissors

pushed through the hole in the skin at an angle of about 45° so that the vein is penetrated close to the skin puncture. Once the tips of both catheter and needle are in the vein, as demonstrated by the presence of blood in the 'flashback' chamber of the catheter (*Fig.* 8.6), the needle is withdrawn a few millimetres within the catheter so that the point is protected by the catheter. The catheter can then be advanced into the vein up to the hub without danger of the needle piercing the vessel wall. The needle is removed and the catheter flushed through with heparinized saline before the end is sealed or injection or infusion

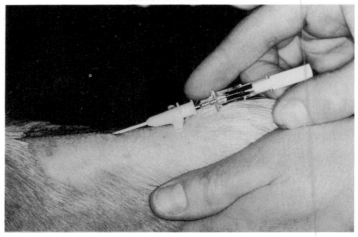

*Fig.* 8.6. The needle has been withdrawn slightly before the cannula is advanced up the vein. Note the presence of blood in the 'flashback' chamber.

started. A cephalic cannula is most easily secured with adhesive tape wound round the leg (*Fig.* 8.7) and should then be bandaged for protection (*Fig.* 8.8).

Jugular catheterization (catheterization implies that the implanted tube is longer than a cannula) should be performed under proper aseptic conditions. The animal is restrained on its side with the neck arched over a small sand bag (*Fig.* 8.9). The vein is then raised by pressure applied in the jugular groove and venepuncture performed as with the cephalic vein, with the catheter directed towards the heart. A long catheter is required for jugular use, and the 'over the needle' type are less suitable since they are not flexible until the needle has been removed. The Deseret 'E-Z cath' has a wire attached to a relatively short needle and has been found satisfactory for jugular catheterization in most dogs. Standard 'over the needle' cannulae are usually adequate for cats. The jugular catheter should not be pushed in right up to the hub. The hub–shaft junction is the weakest point and if it breaks the catheter will be lost into the circulation where it may cause damage to the right side of the heart. The catheter is best secured by suturing it so that 3–6 cm remains outside the skin (*Fig.* 8.10). In the severely collapsed animal it may be necessary to cut down on to the jugular vein in order to locate it. This is a full surgical procedure and must be performed under strict asepsis.

### Cardiopulmonary resuscitation

To be successful, cardiopulmonary resuscitation must be initiated

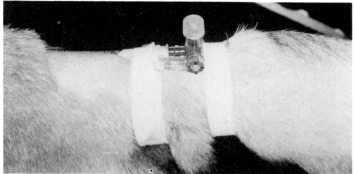

*Fig.* 8.7. The cannula is secured to the leg with two pieces of adhesive tape. The proximal tape is initially taken around the limb before including the cannula hub in the second turn. The distal tape includes the leg and the distal port of the three-way stopcock.

immediately cardiac arrest occurs and must be aggressive. Practice or hospital emergency treatment should be discussed and an agreed course of action drawn up so that there is no confusion or panic when such treatment is required. Effective cardiopulmonary resuscitation requires at least two people; three or four is not excessive as the exhausting cardiac massage is best taken in rotation. The necessary equipment (*Table* 8.3) should be kept together in an easily accessible box. Its contents must be checked regularly so that it can be relied upon in an emergency.

The aim of cardiopulmonary resuscitation is to maintain vital oxygenation and circulation while drugs or other treatment are given to restore the animal's own cardiac and respiratory function. The ABC approach is well tested and is easy to remember in an emergency (*see Table* 8.4).

A — airway — indicates that the first requirement is to establish a clear airway through which oxygen or air can be administered in order to inflate the lungs. This virtually always means than an endotracheal tube must be passed. If airway obstruction is itself the cause of the arrest an emergency tracheostomy may be required (*see below* Tracheostomy).

B — breathing — means that intermittent positive pressure ventilation must be performed (Chapter 1). Ideally this should be with 100 per cent oxygen; air may be used if oxygen supplementation is unavailable. Respiratory rate should be appropriate to the animal concerned: 12/min is suitable for most dogs and 20/min for cats.

C — circulation — means that cardiac massage must be performed to maintain cardiac output. It is essential that the animal is turned on to its side and a pad such as a small sandbag placed under the chest. Firm intermittent pressure is then applied to the chest wall as sharp thumps:

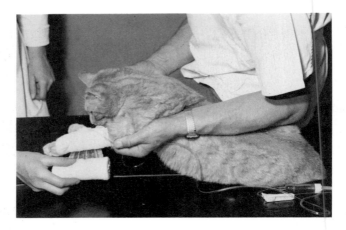

*a*

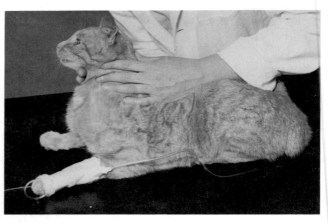

*b*

*Fig.* 8.8. An intravenous cannula bandaged to a cat's leg. *a*, The bandage is taken around the drip extension tubing to prevent the catheter from being pulled out. *b*, The tubing is further secured by the zinc oxide tape.

60 beats per minute is adequate and must be coordinated with respiration. Detection of a femoral pulse, however weak, indicates that the cardiac massage is effective. If effective cardiac massage cannot be performed externally, the chest must be opened and the

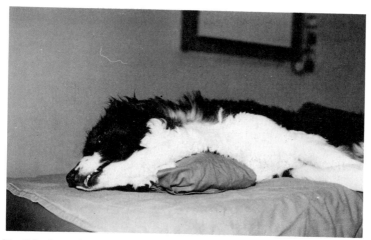

*Fig.* 8.9. A sandbag placed under the dog's neck will aid jugular catheterization.

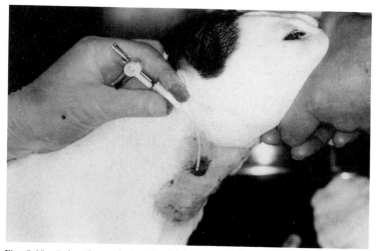

*Fig.* 8.10. A jugular catheter should be secured by suturing in the position shown. The hub and three-way stopcock should also be sutured to the skin to provide additional anchorage.

Table 8.3. *Equipment for cardiopulmonary resuscitation*

| | | |
|---|---|---|
| Endotracheal tubes and connectors | | |
| Oxygen and means of supplying IPPV | | |
| Small sandbag or pad | | |
| Adrenaline | 1:1000 | 1 ml vials |
| Sodium bicarbonate | 5% | 10 ml vials |
| Calcium chloride | 10% | 10 ml vials |
| Lignocaine | 2% | 5 and 20 ml vials (or 50 ml bottle) |
| Atropine | 0·6 mg/ml | 1 ml vials |
| Dobutamine | Vials of 250 mg powder | |
| Syringes (10 ml and 2·5 ml), needles (23 G, 21 G, 20 G and 19 G) | | |
| ECG needles or clips | | |
| File | | |
| Saline or water for injection | | 100 ml bottles |

heart squeezed directly. No time can be wasted in surgical preparation, although wetting the coat over the ribs may help to ensure that a clean cut can be made between two ribs over the heart. If resuscitation is successful, time can be spent later in cleaning and repairing the thoracotomy incision.

Once adequate ventilation and circulation is established thought can be spared for the cause of the arrest and thus rational treatment. In many cases simply reoxygenating the patient is successful. However, where the heart does not begin to beat spontaneously it should be established whether asystole or ventricular fibrillation is present, ideally by connecting an ECG. A defibrillator is required to treat ventricular fibrillation, but if unavailable, adrenaline followed by lignocaine may be successful. Atropine should be administered to remove vagal inhibition, particularly if bradycardia preceded the arrest. Adrenaline is the treatment of choice for asystole, and calcium chloride may be given to improve cardiac contractility. Some degree of cardiogenic shock is likely and administration of fluids and bicarbonate is rational (Chapters 2 and 7). Once sinus rhythm has been established the heart can be supported with a catecholamine drip of either dopamine or dobutamine (Chapters 2 and 7).

## Placing a chest drain

An indwelling pleural drainage tube is required whenever air or fluid is to be removed from the pleural cavity. A small intravenous cannula may be used in an emergency for a single aspiration (*Fig.* 8.11).

The chest wall is clipped and prepared as for surgery. An intradermal injection of local anaesthetic is made over the ninth rib and the needle advanced so that the subcutaneous tissues, intercostal

*Table 8.4.* **Cardiopulmonary resuscitation (CPR)**

---

Call for help
Note the time
A — establish clear airway
B — ventilate 12–20 per min
C — start external cardiac massage
      sandbag under chest
      60 per min
      coordinate with IPPV
    if external massage inadequate, open chest
D — drugs
      establish cause
      connect ECG
      establish i.v. access and give fluids (Ringer's
    lactate)

*Asystole*
Adrenaline
1·0 ml of 1:1000 diluted
  to 10 ml (1:10 000)
i.v., intracardiac or down ET tube
  1–5 ml every 5 min

Calcium chloride
2·5–5 ml of 10% i.v. or intracardiac every 10 min

Atropine
if bradycardia preceded arrest 0·3–0·6 mg i.v.
  (0·5–1·0 ml of 0·6 mg/ml)
Sodium bicarbonate
  as for fibrillation

*Fibrillation*
Adrenaline
  as for asystole

then open chest
Electrical defibrillation

Calcium chloride
  as for asystole

Lignocaine
2·5–5 ml of 2% i.v. bolus

Sodium bicarbonate
1 mmol (mEq)/kg
i.v.
(5% contains 0·6 mmol (mEq)/ml
8% contains 1·0 mmol (mEq)/ml)

Once sinus rhythm established
support with *dobutamine* drip:
  add 10 ml water to 250 mg powder
  add this to 1 litre 5% dextrose
  give 1 drop kg$^{-1}$ min$^{-1}$ (0·04 mg kg$^{-1}$ min$^{-1}$)
or *adrenaline* drip
  dilute 1·0 ml 1:1000 to 50 ml (= 1:50 000)
  give to effect
Monitor ECG and pulse
if *lignocaine* drip required
  500 mg (25 ml of 2%) in 500 ml 5% dextrose
  1–3 ml/min

---

muscle and pleura of the eighth intercostal space are infiltrated. A 14–22 G 'over the needle' cannula is used, depending upon the size of the animal. As soon as the thoracic cavity is penetrated the needle is removed and a syringe and three-way stop cock are quickly attached to the end of the catheter.

Where repeated aspiration is required, more substantial equipment

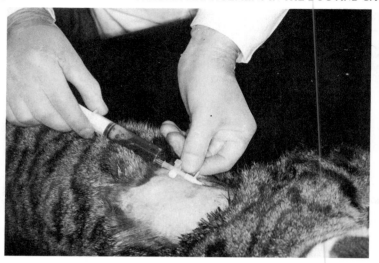

*Fig.* 8.11. An intravenous catheter with three-way stopcock and syringe can be used to aspirate the chest. A larger chest drain is more suitable for long term drainage.

is needed. The lumen of the tubing is easily blocked with blood clots and proteinaceous secretions, and should thus have as large an internal diameter as the size of the animal permits. The tube must also be long enough for a substantial proportion to remain in the pleural cavity in order to prevent accidental displacement. A needle should never be used to aspirate the pleural cavity as there is a danger that the lung tissue may be sliced with the sharp bevel.

A chest drain provides a potentially lethal entry into the pleural cavity. If it is opened to the air a pneumothorax will result. It is essential that the end is always sealed when not connected to a one-way valve or suction. Complete asepsis is also required both in the insertion of the drain and in its management.

Commercially available polythene chest drains (4 and 5 mm internal diameter) supplied with a trocar for insertion (*Fig.* 8.12) have been found satisfactory for both dogs and cats. They produce little tissue irritation and appear less painful than red rubber tubing.

In the dog and cat the most satisfactory point of entry for the tube is between the eighth and ninth ribs approximately two-thirds of the way up the chest wall. A more ventral and anterior approach is preferred by some for fluid drainage. However, the tip of the tube can be positioned according to the area to be drained, and the more caudal approach avoids vital intrathoracic structures.

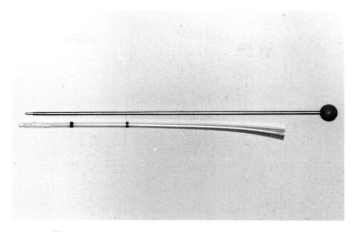

*Fig.* 8.12. An Argyl polythene chest drain and trocar.

*Table 8.5.* **Equipment for placing a chest drain**

Skin prep. (e.g. organic iodine)
Surgical spirit
Local anaesthetic (2% lignocaine)
Syringe and needles
Swabs
Sterile drapes
Suture material (sterile monofilament nylon and
    needle)
Chest drain or large i.v. catheter
Underwater seal bottle and tubing
Means of suction
Clamps and tough suture material to seal drain

Ideally, the necessary equipment (*Table* 8.5) is kept ready in a
sterile pack. The patient is restrained on its side and the site prepared
as for surgery. The area should be draped and sterile gloves used. An
intradermal injection of local anaesthetic is made over the ninth rib
and the resulting weal then pushed forwards so that it lies over the
eighth intercostal space. Local anaesthetic solution is injected into the
intercostal muscles and the underlying pleura. A small incision is made
in the skin through the weal. Two sutures are laid. One is to secure the
tube after it is inserted, the second to close the skin incision when the
tube is removed. With the skin incision held directly over the
desensitized intercostal space, the tubing, with trocar in place, is

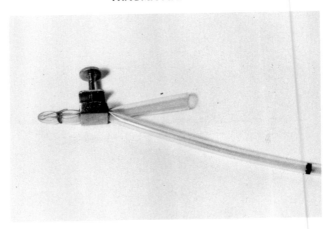

*Fig.* 8.13. The end of the chest drain should be securely closed when not attached to a one-way valve. A gate clamp and suture provide an adequate seal.

inserted into the thoracic cavity through the desensitized tissues. A firm thrust is required to enter the chest without continuing into underlying lung tissue. The trocar is then removed and the end of the drain sealed immediately with either a finger or by attaching a one-way valve. The skin is released so that the skin incision does not lie directly over the intercostal incision and the tube runs through a small tunnel under the skin. This ensures that no air leaks into the pleural cavity around the tube.

When the tube is not in use for suction or attached to an underwater seal the end should be securely sealed and the whole chest bandaged. It is essential that the chest drain is well protected, both to maintain asepsis and to prevent interference by the animal. A 'belt and braces' approach to sealing the end of the tube is appropriate. A plug or gate clamp is used as the short term seal, but, if the tube is to be left *in situ* for any length of time, the tube should be kinked and secured with strong suture material (*Fig.* 8.13). It is also essential to ensure that when the drain is connected to an underwater seal, the animal remains at least 1·2 m above the trap bottle (*Fig.* 8.14) to prevent water from being aspirated into the chest.

**Urinary catheterization**

Urinary catheterization is often required in the care of traumatized patients. It enables urinary output to be accurately measured, it prevents soiling and skin chapping in the incontinent animal and it

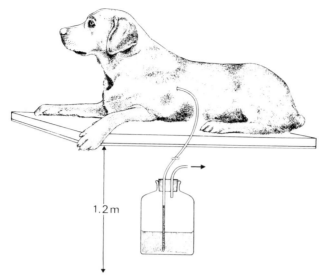

*Fig.* 8.14. The underwater seal must always be kept below the level of the dog or water will be aspirated into the chest.

keeps the bladder empty, thus increasing the animal's comfort and preventing damage caused by over-stretching of the bladder wall.

A self-retaining catheter is the easiest to manage, and the Foley catheter (*Fig.* 8.15), available in 8, 10 and 12 French gauge, is suitable for most bitches. These catheters contain a side channel leading to a balloon at the tip, close to the orifice (*Fig.* 8.16). Once the catheter is in place this balloon is inflated with sterile water so that the tip of the catheter is now too big to be pulled back through the neck of the bladder. Unfortunately Foley catheters are not available for cats, small bitches or male dogs. Jackson cat catheters (*Fig.* 8.17) are available for male cats and can be sutured to the prepuce, but ordinary urinary catheters must be adapted if they are to be left *in situ* in queens and male dogs. This is most easily accomplished by applying a tape 'butterfly' to the catheter which is then sutured to the prepuce or vulva (*Fig.* 8.18).

Urinary catheters should be inserted under aseptic conditions, with the operator wearing sterile gloves. This is particularly important if the catheter is to be left *in situ* for several days. It is most convenient to make up a sterile set (*Table* 8.6) kept ready for the purpose.

To catheterize a male dog the animal is restrained on its side and the penis extruded. The penis and surrounding area is cleaned with organic iodine skin preparation. The tip of the catheter is lubricated

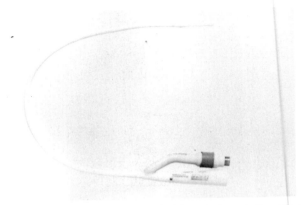

*Fig.* 8.15. Foley catheter. Sterile water is injected through the side arm to inflate the cuff.

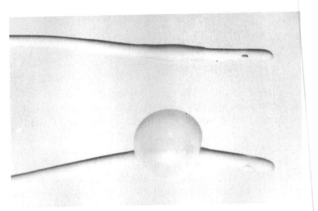

*Fig.* 8.16. Inflated and non-inflated Foley catheters. The inflated bulb prevents the catheter from being pulled out.

and introduced into the urethra. The catheter should be advanced up the urethra firmly but gently. On no account should any force be used as the urethra may easily be damaged or even perforated. The catheter is advanced until a few centimetres (depending on the size of the dog) are within the bladder. Entry into the bladder is usually indicated by passage of urine down the catheter, but occasionally it is necessary to estimate the distance. The catheter is then secured as described above and attached to a urine collection bag (an empty i.v. infusion bag makes an excellent urine collection bag).

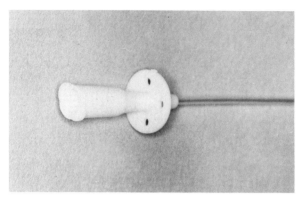

*Fig.* 8.17. Jackson cat catheter. The collar of the catheter can be sutured to the prepuce to prevent it coming out.

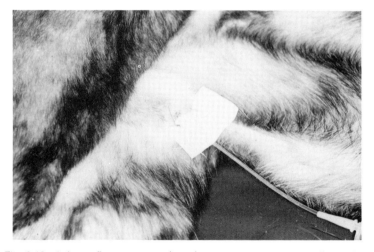

*Fig.* 8.18. A butterfly tape sutured to the prepuce secures an ordinary dog catheter.

The most satisfactory method of catheterizing the bitch is to use a speculum. The bitch is restrained on her back with the hind legs pulled forwards (*Fig.* 8.19). The vulva is cleaned with an organic iodine solution. The speculum is introduced into the vulva with care to avoid the blind ending clitoral fossa. The speculum should be advanced with the tip pointing towards the animal's lumbar spine. The vagina is now

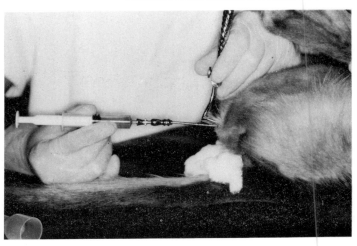

*Fig.* 8.19. The bitch is catheterized in dorsal recumbency with her hindlegs pulled forwards. Once the catheter is in the urethra the legs should be extended.

*Table 8.6. Equipment for inserting urinary catheters*

Organic iodine skin prep.
Sterile lubricant
Swabs
Bitch speculum and light source
Catheters
Sterile saline
Suture material and tape
Urine collection bag

illuminated, ideally with a bulb on the speculum, but if necessary from an outside source. The speculum is adjusted until the urethral orifice can be seen. The catheter is introduced into the orifice and then threaded up the urethra. Once the catheter tip is in the urethra the hind legs can be placed in a more natural position to facilitate the passage of the catheter into the bladder. The Foley catheter is soft and flexible and is most easily inserted with the help of a stiffening wire held in the side holes in the tip of the catheter (*Fig.* 8.20). This is removed after the balloon is inflated. The balloon should not be inflated until the catheter is well into the bladder or it will stretch the urethral wall. The volume of water required to inflate the balloon is indicated on the catheter itself and depends on the catheter gauge. Once the balloon is inflated the catheter can be pulled back so that the balloon rests just inside the neck of the bladder, and a urine collection bag is attached.

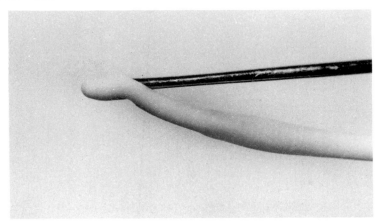

*Fig.* 8.20. A metal probe or stylette facilitates introduction of the soft Foley catheter. The probe is withdrawn from the side hole after the cuff is inflated.

If a suitable speculum is not available, the bitch can be catheterized by palpation. A finger, preferably gloved, is inserted into the vagina, the urethral orifice palpated and the catheter introduced under the guidance of the palpating finger. In the tiny bitch and the queen the vagina is too small for palpation or for a speculum and blind catheterization must be performed. Particular care is required in this instance so that the delicate structures are not damaged.

## Tracheostomy

A tracheostomy may be required to relieve severe upper respiratory tract obstruction. It is also effective in the treatment of intrapulmonary haemorrhage when the tidal volume has been reduced to that of the dead space. Tracheostomy reduces the dead space and thus allows fresh gas to reach the alveoli.

Disposable plastic tracheostomy tubes are commercially available and come in a range of sizes suitable for most dogs and cats (*Fig.* 8.21). These are much more satisfactory than the older metal variety, and can be replaced with a new one whenever necessary.

If an emergency tracheostomy is required, as in a case of complete airway obstruction, speed is of the greatest importance and surgical preparation minimal. However, in many cases there is time for full surgical preparation and this should always be carried out whenever possible.

Tracheostomy is most easily performed with the animal on its back with the head and neck extended. The procedure can be performed under local anaesthesia if necessary. A midline incision is made

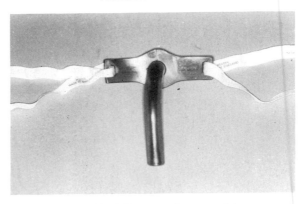

*Fig.* 8.21. A Portex tracheostomy tube.

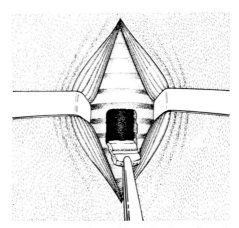

*Fig.* 8.22. Tracheostomy performed by reflecting a flap of tracheal wall.

immediately behind the cricoid cartilage, and the underlying sterno-hyoideus muscles are divided to expose the trachea. Two or three tracheal rings are severed so that a flap can be reflected (*Fig.* 8.22). An appropriate tracheostomy tube is then threaded into the trachea towards the chest, and the tape tied around the animal's neck to secure the tube in place. When the tube is removed, the flap of trachea is repositioned and the overlying tissues sutured. It rarely causes stenosis or presents any problem in healing.

Once a tracheostomy has been performed, the veterinarian and nursing staff are committed to maintaining a clear airway. Without this

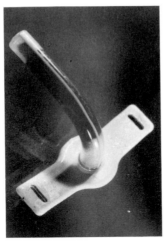

*Fig.* 8.23. A blocked tracheostomy tube may have fatal consequences. The tube must be flushed and aspirated every few hours.

the tube may become blocked, and, since this is now the only airway, an obstructed tracheostomy tube will be fatal (*Fig.* 8.23).

### Intranasal catheter for oxygen administration

Supplementary oxygen is often beneficial in the animal with chest injuries and in shock. However, a mask is often resented and may be counter-productive as oxygen consumption increases when the animal actively resists the mask. A nasal catheter is usually better tolerated and is a viable alternative.

A thin-walled rubber or plastic catheter is lubricated with local anaesthetic gel (e.g. 2 per cent lignocaine) and introduced up the nose until its tip lies in the nasopharynx. To ensure that the correct length of catheter is inserted it should be pre-measured, the tip being level with the angle of the mandible. The catheter is then taped to the nose and connected to the oxygen supply. It is essential that the catheter does not fit tightly in the nostril so that there is no obstruction to breathing. A flow of 1–4 l/min, according to the size of the animal, is generally adequate for most dogs and cats.

### Central venous pressure

Measurement of the central venous pressure provides information about the degree of filling of the vascular bed and also about the cardiac reserve (of the right side of the heart). In effect, it indicates the balance between venous return and cardiac output.

Central venous pressure is measured in the anterior vena cava close to the right atrium. A jugular catheter, 20–30 cm for dogs, or 10–15 cm for cats, is inserted and the tip advanced until it is in the thorax. This is judged both by pre-measuring the catheter and also by the fact that when the catheter tip is in the chest small oscillations in the fluid–air junction are seen with respiration. The jugular catheter is secured in the usual manner and a giving set extension tube, sealed with a three-way stopcock, is connected. An open ended tube (e.g. another giving set extension tube) is joined to one port of the three-way stopcock, and an infusion line from a giving set supplying intravenous fluid is attached to the other port. All the tubing is filled with saline or other crystalloid fluid. A scale in centimetres is fixed beside the open ended tube as this forms the water manometer (*Fig. 8.24*).

The scale zero should be level with the right atrium. It is most convenient to have an external reference point, usually taken as the manubrium as this is readily identifiable for repeated readings. It is important that there is a loop of fluid-filled tubing between the manometer zero and the jugular catheter. This will prevent air entering the vein should central venous pressure be below zero.

To measure central venous pressure the stopcock is turned so that

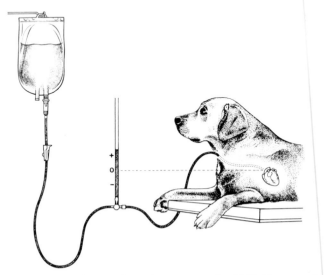

*Fig.* 8.24. A water manometer is used to measure the CVP. The zero of the scale is adjusted to the level of the right atrium.

the manometer tubing is filled from the infusion set. The stopcock is then turned so that the jugular catheter is connected to the manometer and the infusion is switched off. The column of water in the manometer line is then allowed to equilibrate with the venous pressure and the height of the column is measured. This gives the central venous pressure in centimetres of water. A small swing is seen with respiration. Intravenous fluid infusion can be continued between measurements by turning the stopcock to close off the manometer.

Normal central venous pressure is approximately 5 cm $H_2O$. However, since it is difficult to ensure that the same zero point is used on different animals, single readings are of little value and serial readings are much more informative. Observation of the central venous pressure response to a short period of fast infusion (*see* Chapter 7) provides the most useful information as it assesses the ability of the heart to increase its output in response to an increased pre load. If there is little or only a transient increase in central venous pressure in response to this fast infusion, it indicates that the vascular bed is not filled and more fluids should be infused. If there is an increase which is sustained, fluid infusion should be slowed or stopped as it indicates that either the vascular bed is adequately filled or that the heart is unable to increase its output. Other clinical signs must be used to differentiate these conditions.

Simultaneous measurement of arterial blood pressure is the most useful adjunct to central venous pressure as it provides information about the after load. High central venous pressure and low arterial pressure indicates failure of the pump whereas when both are low, fluid deficit is present.

**Arterial catheterization**

Arterial catheterization is rarely performed in small animal practice. However, measurement of arterial blood pressure and arterial blood gas tensions provides valuable information, and can be extremely worthwhile, particularly in the intensive care patient.

The femoral artery is commonly used, but the anterior tibial is an excellent alternative in the larger breeds of dog. In principle, arterial catheterization is similar to venous catheterization. Strict asepsis is required. The vessel is located by palpation of the pulse rather than by direct observation. Once the catheter is in place, and secured by suture or tape, it is sealed with a stopcock or plug and flushed regularly with heparinized saline. Where an anaeroid manometer is used for measurement of mean arterial pressure this is connected to the arterial line with saline filled tubing. It is essential that fluid does not enter the manometer itself. This is avoided either by interposing a column of air or by using a flexible diaphragm as in the Pressurveil system (see *Fig.* 7.7).

When the catheter is removed, firm pressure must be applied to the artery to prevent the formation of a haematoma. Pressure must be maintained for at least 2 minutes, and sometimes 5 or even 10 minutes are required to ensure that bleeding stops. Such pressure is required even when a fine (25 SWG) needle is used for taking arterial blood samples.

### Abdominal paracentesis

Abdominal paracentesis may demonstrate the presence of free fluid within the abdomen but it will not detect damage to the retroperitoneal structures. Blood, urine, bile or intestinal contents may be obtained, but unfortunately a significant number of false negatives occur. Exploratory laparotomy should be performed when the diagnosis is uncertain.

Paracentesis is performed under local anaesthesia with the animal restrained in lateral recumbency. Larger dogs can be kept standing. The skin and underlying body wall is infiltrated with local anaesthetic solution in the midline, just caudal to the umbilicus. A large gauge needle (18–14 SWG) is introduced through the linea alba in the desensitized area. If no drops of fluid appear at the needle hub, gentle aspiration with a syringe should be attempted and the needle can be carefully redirected within the abdomen. It may also be helpful to change the animal's position from lateral recumbency to standing, and to introduce another needle posterior to the first.

### Measurement of packed cell volume and plasma proteins

Packed cell volume (PCV) and plasma protein (PP) concentration are the most useful and straightforward laboratory investigations to perform in order to assess dehydration and monitor fluid therapy.

PCV denotes the relative proportion of cells and plasma in a blood sample, expressed as cell volume as a percentage of the whole. It is a useful index of the effective red blood cell mass and closely correlates with haemoglobin concentration.

The microhaematocrit method is well suited for small animal work. A microhaematocrit centrifuge (*Fig.* 8.25), capillary tubes and a means of sealing the end are required. A glass capillary tube is filled with blood that has been collected into anticoagulant (preferably EDTA). Heparin-coated tubes are also available which can be used for untreated blood. The tip of the tube is sealed with a plasticine plug or by heating it in a Bunsen flame, and the tube is centrifuged at 11 000 rpm for 5 minutes. The relative proportion of cells to plasma is most easily

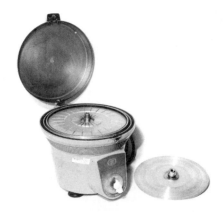

*Fig.* 8.25. A microhaematocrit centrifuge. The blood tubes should be centrifuged at 11 000 r.p.m. for 5 minutes.

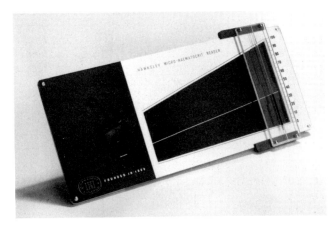

*Fig.* 8.26. A microhaematocrit reader is used to measure the PCV. The tube is positioned so that the total length of the column corresponds to 100 per cent. The sliding marker is adjusted to the cell/plasma interface and the PCV read.

calculated by using a specially designed reader (*Fig.* 8.26), or the height of the column of cells and that of the whole sample is measured and the PCV calculated as follows:

$$\frac{\text{height of cells (cm)}}{\text{height of whole column (cm)}} \times 100$$

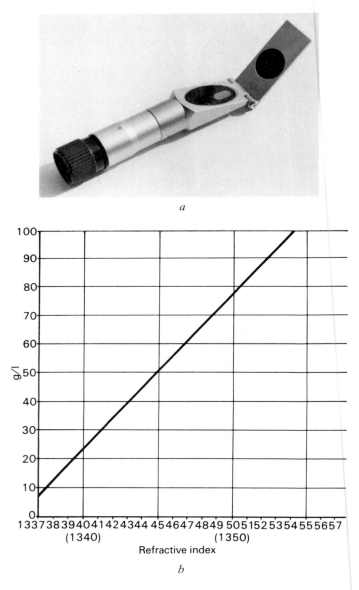

*Fig.* 8.27. *a*, A typical refractometer suitable for measurement of plasma protein concentration. *b*, Conversion from refractive index to plasma protein concentration. (*b*, Reproduced by permission of the Cambridge University Department of Clinical Veterinary Medicine, Clinical Pathology Laboratory.)

The concentration of the proteins in plasma is the main determinant of the refractive index and can thus be measured with a refractometer (*Fig.* 8.27). Lipids, bilirubin and free haemoglobin also contribute to the total solids and influence the refractive index, but an accurate measure of plasma protein is obtained if the plasma is clear.

Clinical refractometers are relatively cheap, easily maintained and are easy to use. The refractive index scale makes it possible for the refractometer to be used for a variety of purposes such as the measurement of specific gravity of urine and other body fluids. An added advantage is the small amount of fluid required (a few drops) for any measurement.

If the microhaematocrit method is used for PCV estimation, an adequate sample of plasma for the refractometer is obtained by scoring and breaking the capillary tube just above the level of the packed cell column. The refractometer is calibrated by applying a drop of distilled water to the clean surface of the test chamber. The refractometer is illuminated (the small portable type is held up to the light) and the scale adjusted so that the line produced is at zero. The plasma sample is then placed on to the sampling chamber, after it has been wiped dry, and the reading taken at the level of the new line that is produced.

## Excretory urography (intravenous urography)

Excretory urography is a useful technique for evaluating the site and extent of injury to the urinary system. Under normal circumstances the patient should be starved for 24 hours and given an enema before the procedure. This is impractical in the trauma case, and some superimposition of ingesta-filled bowel and contrast-filled structures has to be accepted.

The procedure is most easily carried out in the anaesthetized patient. Plain lateral and ventrodorsal radiographs of the abdomen should be taken first. A non-ionic water-soluble iodine solution containing 300 mg I/ml (Omnipaque, Nyegaard Ltd) is used as the contrast agent, given via an intravenous catheter. The pulse should be monitored and, provided it is stable, the contrast agent injected as quickly as possible. Generally a total dose of 800 mg I/kg is given over 2 minutes.

Radiographs are taken immediately after completion of the injection and at 2, 5 and 10 minutes. The contrast-filled renal parenchyma is usually seen on the immediate and 2 minute films, while ureters and bladder are seen at 5 and 10 minutes. Contrast persists for approximately 20 minutes with this technique. If the integrity of the bladder is in doubt, further films taken during this time help to confirm or refute this.

# Equipment and Suppliers

## Urinary catheterization

Foley catheters — Willingtons Medicals Ltd
Jackson cat catheters — All
Disposable cat, dog and bitch catheters } — veterinary suppliers
Vaginal speculum } — Holborn Surgical Instrument Co. Ltd
Metal bitch catheter }

## Intravenous catheters

Cathlon (Critikon Canada Inc.) — Willingtons Medicals Ltd
— W & J Dunlop Ltd
Angiocath (Deseret) } — Beckton Dickinson (UK) Ltd
E–Z Cath (Deseret) }

## Intravenous equipment

Avon giving sets and drip extension tubing } — All veterinary suppliers
Three-way stopcocks } — Vygon (UK) Ltd
Catheter plugs }
Blood collection packs: Fenwal (Travenol) } — Travenol Laboratories Ltd
— Arnolds Veterinary Supplies Ltd
Tuta (Cutter Laboratories) — Miles Laboratories Ltd

## Chest drains etc.

Argyl chest drains } — Arnolds Veterinary Products Ltd
Tracheostomy tubes (Portex) }
Underwater seal (bottle and tubing) — G.U. Manufacturing Co. Ltd
Heimlich valve — Willingtons Medicals Ltd

147

## Bandages

Elasticated
  Vetrap (3M)
  Elastoplast (Smith & Nephew)
  Treatplast (Vet. Drug Co.)

All veterinary suppliers

  Co-Form/Co-Lastic/Co-Ripwrap (Millpledge)

Millpledge Pharmaceuticals.

Conforming:
  Kling (Johnson & Johnson)

All veterinary suppliers

  Vet-K-Band (Millpledge)

Millpledge Pharmaceuticals

Orthopaedic padding
  Velband (Johnson & Johnson)
  Soffban (Smith & Nephew)

All veterinary suppliers

## Splints

Plastic orthopaedic splints
Zimmer orthopaedic splints

Arnolds Veterinary Products Ltd

## Blankets and insulation

Vetbed — All veterinary suppliers
Plastic bubbles — Any large stationery suppliers

## Laboratory equipment

Refractometer
Microhaematocrit centrifuge

Arnolds Veterinary Products Ltd

Microhaematocrit reader — Hawksley and Sons Ltd

## Suture materials

Dexon (Davis & Geck)
Vicryl (Ethicon)

Macarthys Surgical Ltd
All veterinary suppliers

## Anaesthesia and oxygen administration

| | |
|---|---|
| Ambu bag | Ambu International (UK) Ltd |
| Laryngoscope Soper blade (child for dogs, baby for cats) | Penlon Ltd |
| Halls mask<br>Nasal tube (stomach tube)<br>Magill endotracheal tubes | Arnolds Veterinary Products Ltd and all Veterinary suppliers |
| Ayre's T-piece | Arnolds Veterinary Products Ltd |
| Water's Cannister<br>Two stage oxygen reducing valve | Arnolds Veterinary Products Ltd and Bowring Engineering |

## Intravenous fluids

| | |
|---|---|
| Electrolyte solutions<br>Haemaccel (Hoechst) | All veterinary suppliers |
| Amino acid solutions with or without glucose and fructose: Vamin (Kabivitrum)<br>Fat emulsion: Intralipid (Kabivitrum) | Willingtons Medicals Ltd |
| Sodium bicarbonate<br>Polyfusor (Boots)<br>($8\cdot4\% = 1$ mmol (mEq/l)<br>($4\cdot2\% = 0\cdot5$ mmol (mEq/l)<br>Potassium chloride<br>(20–30 mmol (mEq/l)<br>5 and 10 ml ampoules | Try local pharmacy (dispensing chemist) preferably the smaller private firms. Also local hospital or GP may help |

## Arterial blood pressure measurement

| | |
|---|---|
| Pressurveil anaeroid manometer | Henley's Medical Supplies Ltd |
| Indirect blood pressure monitor: Parkes (model 811) ultrasonic Doppler flow detector | Parkes Electronics (USA) |

## Radiographic contrast material

| | |
|---|---|
| Omnipaque (Nyegaard Ltd) | Nyegaard Ltd |

## ADDRESSES

Arnolds Veterinary Products Ltd
14 Tessa Road
Richfield Avenue
Reading
Berks
RG1 8NF
(0734) 54064

Ambu International (UK) Ltd
Charlton Road
Midsomer Norton
Bath
BA3 4DR
(0761) 416868

Beckton Dickinson (UK) Ltd
Between Towns Road
Cowley
Oxford
OX4 3LY
(0865) 777722

Bowring Engineering
Unit 14, Crawley Mill
Witney
Oxford
OX8 5TJ
(0993) 4025

Centaur Services Ltd
Centaur House
Torbay Road
Castle Cary
Somerset
DG1 2QD
(0963) 50428

Davis & Geck
Fareham Road
Gosport
Hants
PO13 0AS
(0329) 236131

W & J Dunlop Ltd
Veterinary Division
1–9 St Michael's Street
Dumfries
DG1 2QD
(0387) 63733

Ethicon Ltd
P.O. Box 408
Bankhead Avenue
Edinburgh
EH11 4HE
031 453 5555

G.U. Manufacturing Co. Ltd
Plympton St
London
NW8 8AB
01 723 9287

Hawksley and Sons Ltd
Peter Road
Lancing
Sussex
BN15 8TN
(0903) 752815

Henley's Medical Supplies Ltd
Clarendon Road
Hornsey
London N8 0DL
01 889 3151

Holborn Surgical Co. Ltd
Dolphin Works
Margate Road
Broadstairs
Kent
CT10 2QQ
(0843) 61418

Macarthy's Surgical Ltd
Selinas House
Dagenham
Essex
RM8 1QD
01 593 7511

Miles Laboratories Ltd
PO Box 37
Stoke Poges
Slough
SL2 4LY
(02814) 5151

Millpledge Pharmaceuticals
Whinleys Estate
Church Lane
Clarborough
Notts
DN 22 9NA
(0777) 705142

Nyegaard (UK) Ltd
Nycomed House
2111 Coventry Road
Sheldon
Birmingham
B26 3EA
021 742 8781

Parkes Electronics
PO Box 5669
Beaverton
Aloha
Oregon 97006
USA

Penlon Ltd
Abingdon
Oxford
OX14 3PH
(0235) 24042

Travenol Laboratories
Stephenson Way
Thetford
Norfolk
IT24 3SE
(0842) 5911

Veterinary Drug Co. Ltd
Common Road
Dunnington
York
YO1 5RU
(0904) 48844

Vygon (UK) Ltd
Bridge Road
Cirencester
Glos.
GL7 1PT
(0285) 67051

Willingtons Medicals Ltd
Lancaster Road
Shrewsbury
Shropshire
SY1 3NX
(0743) 60244

Every effort has been made to ensure that the above information was correct at the time of going to press. We apologize to any suppliers who may have been omitted.

# Bibliography

Arnoczky S. P. and Greiner T. P. (ed.) (1979) Surgical techniques. *Vet. Clin. North Am. (Small Anim. Pract.)* **9**, no. 2.

Brinker W. O., Piermattei D. L. and Flo G. L. (1983) *Handbook of Small Animal Orthopaedics and Fracture Treatment.* Philadelphia, Saunders.

Burrows C. F. (1981) Veterinary intensive care. *J. Small Anim. Pract.* **22**, 231–52.

Crane S. W. (ed.) (1980) Trauma. *Vet. Clin. North Am. (Small Anim. Pract.)* **10**, no. 3.

Denny H. (1986) Acute trauma in small animals: 3, Orthopaedic injuries. *In Practice* **8**, 168–175.

Foster J. (1985) Acute trauma in small animals: 1. Initial assessment and management. *In Practice* **7**, 173–81.

Herrtage M. E. and Carr L. (1986) Urine sampling in the bitch. *In Practice* **8**, 221–234.

Hickman J. and Walker R. G. (1980) *An Atlas of Veterinary Surgery.* Bristol, Wright.

Hoerlein B. F. (1978) *Canine Neurology: Diagnosis and Treatment.* Philadelphia, Saunders.

Houlton J. E. F. (1986) Acute trauma in small animals: 2, Thoracic injuries. *In Practice* **8**, 152–161.

Kirk R. W. and Bistner S. I. (1981) *Handbook of Veterinary Procedures and Emergency Treatment*, 3rd ed. Philadelphia, Saunders.

Michel A. R. (1985) What is shock? *J. Small Anim. Pract.* **26**, 719–38.

Wingfield W. E. (1981) Emergency medicine. *Vet. Clin. North Am (Small Anim. Pract.)* **11**, no. 1.

# Index